SOLUTIONS FOR HEALTHCARE

Dr. David Bush's new book has the potential to save people a lot of money by eliminating needless doctor visits and save lives by warning us when we should see a doctor now! Having been his patient for over 15 years I know David continually explores and practices proven, leading edge medical techniques to deliver the very best, informed advice to us. I recommend everyone read this outstanding book and keep it within easy reach!

Jed Niederer ~ author of the Best-selling book *Coach Anyone About Anything* and performance coach to companies around the world.

SOLUTIONS FOR HEALTHCARE

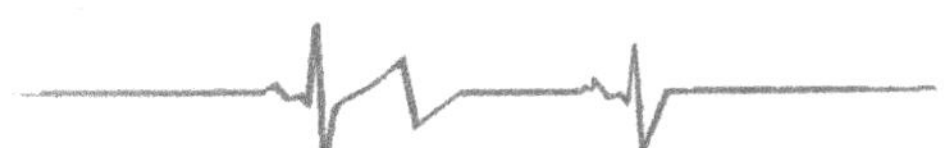

How to avoid doctor visits or know you have to go

ISBN-10: 0986125482
ISBN-13: 978-0-9861254-8-5

DEDICATION

I dedicate this book to my wife, Dawn, who loves me even when I don't deserve love. To my children, Jaclyn and Savana, who gave me renewed purpose. To my family and friends who have inspired me when inspiration was hard to find and to Jed and Germaine for excellent vision and advice when I felt "blocked".

I also dedicate this book to everyone who has ever gone to the doctor and asked the question, "How did this happen to me?" My great hope and wish for you is that this book might give you the knowledge to achieve all you dream of, a plan to make your dreams come true, and the passion to live as great a life as you can.

ACKNOWLEDGMENTS

There are too many people to acknowledge to list them all here. If you have ever written anything of substance about health or healthcare, consider this acknowledgment for you. I took information and content from many places and in many forms to compose this book. Most of the ideas herein are from internet websites which all contain complex ideas written for people who are searching for simple solutions to complex questions. Thank you all for giving me a place to start!

Table of Contents

INTRODUCTION

If you have ever been to the doctor or a hospital, you know one thing for sure. Our health care system in the United States doesn't work very well.

In fact, there is a recent study done by a medical doctor which stated that of the 13 major countries in the world, the United States is 13th!

The main reasons for the poor ranking are the way we are all taught to use healthcare, and the controlling factors that regulate the delivery of healthcare in the U.S.

Healthcare in the U.S. is delivered in such a way that it forces the patient into a critical problem before they ever get to the doctor's office. Many doctors today are forced to practice medicine by making the patient choose what they treat, and measuring the outcome of the treatment rather than treating the cause of the disease. This is like playing cards with a dealer who stacks the deck on every hand. It has taken the art of medicine and made most encounters into a business transaction with very little regard for the needs of the patient.

I wrote this book for a very specific reason… I believe that everyone has the right to the best healthcare they can afford.

I wrote this book for a very specific reason…I believe that everyone has the right to the best healthcare they can afford. Healthcare is one of those things in life that should be immune from outside influences, but the truth is, it is affected by politics and people who abuse it to make money. I wrote this book because I see firsthand every day how frustrated people are with the state of healthcare and how it is delivered.

Even with the advent of the Internet, the information you need gets muddied by people with agendas (good and bad). I believe that if you have the right kind of information, written in terms you can easily understand, you will begin to make small changes in your daily life, which will impact and change your future health for the better.

The real truth is any small change you make when it comes to your health can pay you back in huge ways. Understanding what you can do to control and ***direct your health*** is the foundation you must build on to get healthy. Your future is waiting for you, and I know you can change your life for the better with just a few simple steps.

I hope this book will be a step in the right direction for you and your family. As a doctor, it hurts my heart to see children and people of all ages who have waited too long to avoid preventable effects of disease. They come to me and others like me hoping for a miracle, to be told, "If only…" My wish and desire for you and your family is that **we** will find a way to end disease and suffering on every level. It begins when you understand what to do and **act on the knowledge**.

When I was researching this book, there were thousands of articles that talked about health risks and how they affect the health of people in the United States. The two most dangerous modifiable health risks (things you can control or change all by yourself) are smoking and obesity (being excessively fat). What this means to you is if you smoke and are overweight, you more than double your risks of dying from a related disease ***that is preventable.***

The two most dangerous modifiable health risks… are smoking and obesity….

This is the real reason I wrote this book. My hope is to get people to read and act on the information inside this book and to give the information to other people they care about so there will be less disease in the world.

We ***all know*** that smoking cigarettes can kill you, but some of us still smoke. When I was young, smoking was cool! I admit, I tried every form of tobacco available. I smoked, chewed, dipped and spit myself into more than one headache and stomachache. Luckily for me, I don't do things that make me feel bad for long, so I quit after tobacco made me sick and before I got addicted.

I have also included a lot of information about alternative types of care in each section. These treatments can be used to prevent disease and to help make medical care or therapy more effective.

Please do not think these treatments can be used by themselves as a treatment or cure for any disease a doctor tells you he has diagnosed. Using alternatives like acupuncture, massage, energy medicine or chiropractic to treat a serious medical condition could cause the condition to get much worse. However, there have been many times when we have had patients come in after a surgery only to report, "I don't feel any better now than I did before my surgery."

In the office, I ask all of our patients to get second and even third opinions on any surgery and to find surgeons with no less than an excellent reputation. Surgery is a very serious undertaking because you can never get uncut. With that in mind, I would ask you to take this advice to heart whenever you need surgery. Do your research, and get as much input and information as you can before you get surgery!

I also get a lot of questions about medication. In the past, people had a lot of trust for doctors. You may have been one of those people who never questioned anything your doctor did or told you to do. Today we have the Internet. This means that you can look up the drugs your doctor prescribes for you. You should ***always do this***. Not to question what your doctor is doing, but because every drug has a side effect. If you know what the side effects are before you start taking a drug, then you won't be surprised when they happen.

...one more thing you need to know...is how your medications work together, or what happens if they don't...

There is also one more thing you need to know before you take more than one medication, which is how your medications work together, or what happens if they don't work together. Many people have no idea that some medications don't work well with vitamins or natural remedies or certain foods when taken at the same time.

There is a simple solution that will give you valuable information about how drugs interact or interfere with each other. If you have more than one doctor prescribing drugs for you, you may have been suffering from a drug-drug interaction that creates a side effect you don't want. You can check your drugs and make sure you get what you need, by using a drug interaction checker on the Internet. (http://www.drugs.com/drug_interactions.html)

This brings us to the next important point and one of the **BIG** takeaways you should get from this book. If you don't take care of yourself, no one else will! I have included a number of ways that you can avoid being sick and stay healthy.

The best medicine, in our minds, is no medicine, or as little medicine as you must have for life. When you get older, things don't work as well as they did when you were young. There are many reasons why this is true, but as you take charge of your health, you will find that you can and will get what you want if you know what to ask for.

Why You Must Choose and Focus

The big mistake most people make when they try to improve their health is they don't ask the right questions. They go into the doctor's office with a symptom of a disease or a condition they want the doctor to fix or improve with no idea of what the real problem is and how to ask for help. What you want, what you need to ask for, is how to correct the **root cause** of your condition or disease.

What happens is we all get our focus changed when we first see the doctor. The first question most of us hear when we see the doctor is, "What brought you in today?" We then answer, "I'm here because I feel..." or, "I wanted to find out why I'm having..." These statements automatically start a chain reaction that ends with a treatment that is intended to treat a symptom or a sign of a disease without treating the cause of the disease.

If you do not ask the right questions, the doctor will do what he was trained to do instead of doing what you really ***need him to do***.

If you do not ask the right questions, the doctor will do what he is trained to do instead of doing what you really need him to do.

I want you to get what you want and ***need*** from your healthcare experience. This is the real reason I wrote this book and the reason you should use the information to guide you in the future. You must keep the doctor or the nurse focused, and make sure they don't get distracted when you seek care.

Asking the right questions is the only way this will happen. To ask the right questions, you must understand what is happening, why it is happening, and what your part will be in correcting and preventing the condition or disease.

In order to accomplish this vital and lifesaving goal, you need to understand how your body works on a basic level. Doctors and nurses are trained to treat the symptoms you tell them you want them to treat. They will never guess or try to expand on what you have told them unless they believe that you are not capable of telling them the real problem.

When I was a young boy, probably 12 or 13 years old, I woke up one morning with severe pain. I went in and immediately told my mother that something was wrong. I knew something was wrong because I had groin pain that radiated into my left side. We left immediately and my mother drove me into town.

The only problem was, the farther she drove, the worse my pain got. Even the smallest bump in the road caused severe pain. The pain was so bad I felt like I would throw up or pass out. Eventually, she pulled over and took me to the emergency room where they immediately started to work me up.

As a teenager, I felt that I should just be quiet and let the doctors and nurses do their work. They'd take care of me, I was sure. The problem was, they were looking in the wrong place the whole time. They had just announced to my mother that I was OK, ***and were getting ready to send me home when I knew I had to say something***.

I simply looked at the doctor and I said, "Excuse me, but you're not looking in the right place!" The look on his face was actually a bit intimidating. He thought I was making the whole thing up for attention until I showed him exactly where my pain was and I told him to check my groin. After he did, things went really fast! Within twenty minutes a specialist had me in the operating room and was doing emergency surgery on me.

This is an example of what you must do when you visit the doctor every time. Sometimes, when we are in the doctor's office or the hospital, there are too many distractions for them to make the right call. This could lead to hours of suffering and many times leads to an improper diagnosis and the wrong treatment.

When you use this book and the information inside correctly, you will be armed with ways to make sure that you get the right kind of care and the right amount of care to fix the problem. Getting both is like getting the perfect drink from Starbucks—it doesn't get much better if you love coffee! Not only will you feel better, but you'll actually get better and stay well.

So, what you need is a plan to make sure you get what you want whenever you go to the doctor. This needs to be simple, direct, and it needs to be focused. What happens in a typical doctor-patient interaction is often directed by your complaint, or what the doctor thinks is your complaint.

If you focus the visit on the cause of the complaint, you will get much better results overall. So, you must first understand what the cause is, or may be, and how you need to ask for the right help. Before we go into all of the different types of diseases and the causes, it is important for you to have an understanding of the different types of care and how you should use them.

1

Different Types of Care

There are two main dividing lines in the healing arts, standard medical care (Western medicine) and alternative forms of care (everything else).

You should already be familiar with *Western medicine*. It is probably what you already use for basic, day-to-day health for you and your family. The way this model works is really pretty simple: you get up and you don't feel well, you go to your family doctor and he/she asks you… "So, what brought you in today?"

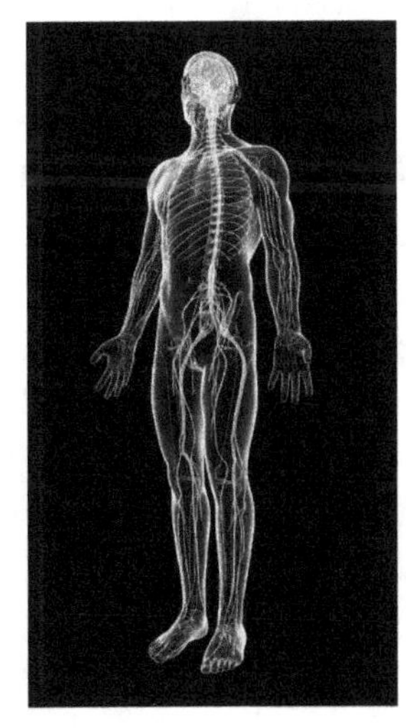

The usual pattern is, when you go to the doctor you are very likely getting some type of medicine, usually a prescription, to treat the first thing you tell the doctor at this point. If you tell him you have a pain, you're going to be treated with a drug or a compound to lessen or get rid of the pain. If you tell him you have a fever or another ***symptom***, you'll get a treatment designed to lessen the discomfort or signs of the disease (which are different from the cause of your symptom) until you begin to get well.

Now, let's take just a minute to examine the last paragraph. It says pretty clearly, as I have mentioned before, that the doctor or the care-giver treats you for what you say is bothering you. This may happen even if you know what the actual problem is, and even worse, ***when you have no idea what the problem is***.

So, Western medicine is designed to treat patients for complaints or symptoms only. If you have an infection, and the doctor can tell you do, they will treat you with an antibiotic or another drug designed to help your body overcome the infection. But, they cannot and will not give you a drug or make you a potion that will make you well. PLEASE understand this vital point!

The other type of care is very simply…everything else. Alternative care is defined as any type of care that is ***not*** traditional medical or Western care! Simply put, it includes chiropractic care, Eastern medicine (which includes acupuncture, acupressure, herbal therapies, magnetic therapy, Qui Gong or energy work, and some other forms of body work), massage, and other forms of healing therapies like naturopathic medicine, nutrition, and the newer type of energy or frequency medicine.

There are literally hundreds of different types of healing therapies that work some of the time for some people. This is why there is so much confusion as to which approach you should or could use to get better! The main difference between the different types of care is the approach used by the caregiver when you go to the office or place of business.

Western medicine is what most of us in the U.S. call standard medical care. This is the largest form of health care rendered world-wide, and you get your care from medical doctors and nurses, osteopathic doctors and physical therapists, and other providers of care.

The doctor will usually ask you what your problem is, and then offer you care that is based around relief of that symptom. They will usually give you drugs of one kind or another or prescribe some sort of therapy to help you get better.

Chiropractic care is the second largest health care profession in the world, but there are far fewer Doctors of Chiropractic (DCs) to provide the care. In some of the more rural areas, this may be a problem because there are more patients per doctor. In this type of care, the Doctor of Chiropractic will use mainly spinal manipulation, which is an adjustment of the bones of the spine (located in your back) to improve the function of the nerve system (the brain and the nervous system).

In this approach, the overall result is not aimed at getting rid of your pain. Instead, the doctor and his staff are trying to get your body to heal itself by removing any interference in your nerve system that could cause pain or disease.

No matter what you may have heard or read, chiropractic is very safe for those who use it. Every year, millions of adjustments are given by Doctors of Chiropractic (DCs) with very few reported injuries or side effects from the adjustment. Chiropractors have one of the lowest costs for malpractice insurance. This is a validation of the safety of the profession.

Eastern medicine and other types of alternative therapies are grouped together, not because they are less important or less effective, but in this book we will consider these providers as a group, because far fewer people look for help from these providers. In this type of care, the approach is again to treat the patient/client for symptoms and the caregiver will use many different types of techniques and/or methods to accomplish this goal.

All of the other therapies are usually not used individually to solve a medical problem, but are used by most people in combination to improve their health and enhance their ability to stay well. If I went in detail into every form of care you could use, this book would simply be too long. So, if you want or need more information about other types of care, just use our good friend Google!

If I went in detail into every form of care you could use, this book would simply be too long.

There are many excellent people in all types of health care. Most of these people are dedicated to helping others, or they wouldn't be in the profession in the first place. That said, if you ever get a feeling that something is wrong, or could be better, please speak up and tell someone in the office! If the situation doesn't get better, leave and find another provider to help you with your problem!

Anyone can do a simple search on the Internet and find hundreds of offers of a cure for any disease, including cancer. So, who or what should you trust? I recommend you trust yourself! Learn the basic methods in this book to get better and stay better for life!

As health care professionals with combined decades of active service to the public in almost all types of care available, my wife and I have a solid foundation in how to get healthy and stay healthy! I can assure you that when one of my family members gets sick, we don't necessarily just do what the first doctor tells us to do!

Once you have all of the facts, you must consider the risks of the treatment offered and determine quickly how you are going to proceed. My wife and I have a plan of action for most of the major diseases (should anyone get sick from cancer, a stroke, or have a heart attack), and we recommend everyone do the same.

Once you have all the facts, you must consider the risks of the treatment offered and determine quickly how you are going to proceed.

What a plan of action does for you and your family is it helps you make critical decisions before you face them and have to deal with the emotions and the disease. Make your plan of action and put it in writing!

For example, after all of my experience in hospitals, witnessing what patients are put through during cancer treatment or recovery from a major heart attack or stroke, I have decided that I do not want excessive measures taken by medical people to save my life.

I have a friend who was a chiropractor in a small city in Texas. He took over his practice when his father had a stroke after serving the community for many years. I went to visit his father in a 24-hour care facility and was shocked to see him lying in bed without help or attention from his caregivers. The truth is, he never got any better after his stroke. I decided then that I didn't want this to be my fate if I should ever have a serious or fatal illness.

Some may consider this to be a cop out, but the last thing I want in my life is to suffer for months after a major illness in order to be bedridden for the rest of my life. If I suffer a serious disease or injury, I don't want that for me or my family!

Use this information to help you design your health care plan for life by deciding what type of health you want. Then pick the ways you will work to get those results. Unfortunately, you cannot have excellent health without the necessary work.

Today a lot of people are getting healthier, but some are just waiting for things to get better and hoping that they will be rescued from themselves. All of the research shows that this is not possible! You ***must take the right action to get what you want from your life!*** We tell our patients every day that if they do small things consistently they can and will change the course and the outcome of their lives in a very big way.

Make a plan and be consistent! This is the only way to get or regain your health!

Make a plan and be consistent! This is the only way to get or regain your health! Now that you understand the basics and the different types of care available, let's get started!

I will give you a description of the most common types of disease and the causes…you get to decide what type of care you would like if you are sick or get sick in the future. Use this book to guide your plans and then take action to stay healthy!

All of the experts agree that prevention is the best way to avoid the expense and the suffering you will be subject to if you lose your health and you get sick. I will give you the best methods available to prevent disease and a comparison of the different treatment types so you can make the decisions you want! Now, let's begin!

2

Use This Book to Create a Better Life!

This book can be the best investment of time and money you ever make if you use it in the right way. I have included in every section the most common reasons people go to the doctor and the simple things you can do to fix health problems before disease starts. The information inside can literally save you thousands, if not hundreds of thousands, of dollars and save you and those you love countless hours of suffering and pain.

This book is written to give you a path to follow that can be easily followed for the rest of your life. This will be a journey for some, but for anyone who makes the choice to follow the instructions, you will be amazed at how much you can and will do to make your life better.

There are sections in the book that deal with different types of health problems. You can turn to the index to find a specific problem or an issue that you may need help with. I have written the book to give you ideas you can use to help a problem; however, as with ***any medical book***, please do not take the information here (or anywhere else you find it) as the only method of treatment, or use it to diagnose a disease or condition. This can be dangerous! If you think you may be sick, ***PLEASE*** get help from a qualified (licensed) medical professional.

This first section is a guide for you to use. Look at the signs of disease. Those are the things you may see or feel when you get sick. And then look for the section that deals specifically with those types of problems. For example, if someone is throwing up, this may be a stomach or digestive problem. There are simple ways to determine which basic problems drive people to the doctor or the hospital.

I will write about different types of problems in simple, everyday language to prevent confusion.

I will write about different types of problems in simple, everyday language to prevent confusion. I am going to give you some simple advice that you may use to help yourself, or someone you know who is sick. These treatments will help the condition or sickness, but they will ***not cure a person who is really sick for a long time***.

If you or someone you love is sick, time is the most critical part of the health equation. Do not let extra minutes pass if you think you or someone else needs help, ***get it now!*** Ask for advice or help or (worst case scenario) dial 9-1-1 as soon as you feel overwhelmed. Waiting could be disastrous!

Some of the sections that deal with different body problems are long and have more details than others. I wrote the book in a specific order to try to discuss the most common complaints we see. Our office is a Family Practice and does not deal with specific conditions like cancer that require a specially trained doctor for care. I will give you advice on how to avoid deadly diseases like cancer and heart-related issues.

One of the questions we hear almost daily in our office from patients is, "Doctor, how did this happen to me?" What everyone wants to know is why they are suffering from the problems that bring them into the office in the first place. The truth is that there is no way for any doctor to know exactly how any person gets sick. There are simply too many things involved in how a person's body works to know exactly what made them sick or how they got sick in the first place.

With that in mind, you need to know that most of the time when you go to the doctor he gives you a diagnosis after he examines you, or he does tests to confirm what he thinks is the problem. Most of the time, a diagnosis is simply a description of what the doctor thinks the problem is, in ***Latin or medical language***.

We have patients come to our office for care and they tell us, "I have sciatica!" or "I have bursitis!" These medical terms are just a description of what you told your doctor was wrong. This is not a way for the doctor to mislead or impress you; it is done because doctors and nurses are taught specific language we all use to clarify conditions and illnesses or diseases.

I will not use those terms in this book. I want you to understand what you have in terms you will understand. If you want more information about a disease or an illness, we have provided hot links (Internet references through the text of the book that will take you to other sites) that will clear up, or, in some cases, further muddy the water for you. When you locate your problem, I suggest that you also look at other sections that may be related. For example, there are a ***lot*** of conditions and illnesses that can be the result of a bad diet.

Action Plan - Getting Started

1. Make a list of all of your symptoms and decide how you want the doctor to help you.
2. Make sure you are clear on the following:
   - how the problem started
   - what makes you feel better or worse?
   - is there a specific time of day or night you feel better or worse?
   - what have you done and did it work (medicines you took are a must)
   - how bad is your problem or pain (scale of 1-10, 10 is worst)?
   - be clear on what you want the doctor to address during the visit
3. Make a list of your other health issues and how you are being treated for those issues, and if the treatment is working well.
4. Make a list of your medicines, list your doses, how many times per day you take the drug, and how long you have been using the drug. Include why you are taking the medicine, if it is working, and if you have any of the side effects from taking the drug.
5. **Get a second (or third) opinion for any surgical recommendation. Only use excellent doctors with great references.**

3

Everything is Connected!

One big point you must understand, which is ***critical and important to your health***, is that everything is connected! We all (well, almost all) know the song about the knee bone's connected to the thigh bone. As silly as the song is, it really is true! Everything is connected and, unfortunately, everything is impacted by everything else when it comes to your (our) health!

Your body is a complex and interconnected living system. Your brain sends out signals that control and coordinate all of your bodily functions. With proper control from the brain and the nerve system, everything in your body will happen at exactly the right time.

Your heart will beat, sending nutrition to every cell in your body; your lungs will fill with oxygen that is transported to all of the cells and tissues by the blood. Waste products of cell function are moved through your body by the blood and the lymph system to the filtration systems of the liver and kidneys. The digestive system will break down food, which is converted into a usable form of energy for the cells, and the waste is moved into the large intestine and bladder out of your body.

All of this and more happens all day every day without any real effort on your part. However, any upset in this delicate, complex and balanced system could lead to a loss of health, disease, and even death!

This is why you must be aware of how important it is for you to become more involved and aware of how much control you have over your health. If you decide that you don't care, or it takes too much effort to make a difference in your health outcomes, then you will get less health in this lifetime! Everything you do has a direct impact on your health!

Everything you do has a direct impact on your health!

We have seen it more than we care to admit. There have been many instances, during every month we have been in health care, when a patient will come in and they are very ill from doing ***one thing*** wrong for a very long time!

Currently, we see an awful lot of people with headaches that won't go away. WHY? Because a lot of people now work with their head down over a computer or a desk all day, and then they go home and do the same thing. Many of us work in positions that are bad for our health. There are even new diseases and conditions that have been created because of these types of problems (IT neck, pocket-book sciatica, and carpal tunnel).

What this means is your body is impacted and ***changed*** by everything you do. If you are forced to do something consistently wrong, it could cost you your health! I remember a particular case I was given when I was in school. A man had a really bad spinal problem, with lots of pain in one leg and a severe limp. When I looked at him on the exam, I found he had one leg that was two inches shorter than the other. I asked him some more questions to try to find out why this happened and the reason was…he stood on one leg all day to work a metal pressing machine at work. He did this for over 20 years!

This man had developed a short leg because he used a pedal all day with one leg and stood all day on the other! His body had actually worn out one side from standing and the result after 20 years was his leg was two inches shorter on one side, which made his spine lean to one side and pinched the nerves in his lower back.

He had no other types of injuries and reported no accidents that would make his condition worse. He simply did the same thing (hundreds of thousands of times) all day and he paid a very steep price for being a loyal, hard-working employee at a machine shop!

Your body knows when you have a fingernail or cuticle that is trimmed wrong. In fact, it will probably bother you endlessly until you fix it!

Your body has a brain that is in complete control all of the time. It keeps your essential functions working perfectly to keep you alive, it takes the food you eat and turns it into usable energy, and it fights off infection and other threats to your health on a minute-by-minute basis!

Your body has a brain that is in complete control all the time.

The brain and the nervous system control and connect all of the body systems. Without your brain working, you simply cannot live!

When I was a child, they used to teach us that our heart was the most important organ in the body. Now we know without question that the brain is the most important organ in the body, and the nerve system (which connects the brain to the body) is a close second!

If you want a real life example of just how important these two systems are, just remember what happened to Christopher Reeve (Hollywood's Superman of movie fame). He was a very good horseman who fell off his horse while trying to make a jump.

The fall caused one injury that was very severe and cost this fine gentleman his life. When he fell, reports show he broke the top bones in his neck, which damaged his spinal cord near the base of his brain. The result was, this man, who was in near-perfect physical shape before the fall, spent the rest of his life in a wheelchair and was paralyzed from the neck down. He eventually died from complications of this injury because his organs began to fail from a lack of nerve system energy from his brain.

...if you ever lose the control and coordination your brain provides, your health will suffer.

This proves a very important point...if you ever lose the control and coordination your brain provides, your health will suffer. Many medical studies and reports support this statement. So this raises another problem: how do you keep your nerve system healthy? Your nerve system is protected by the bones of the spinal column and the discs that serve as cushions between the bones.

You must take care of your spine to prevent a loss of control and/or a loss of function in your nerve system which controls your body. Every single cell in your body depends on the messages that start in your brain, then travel over the spinal cord and nerves. (http://www.nimh.nih.gov/health/educational-resources/brain-basics/brain-basics.shtml)

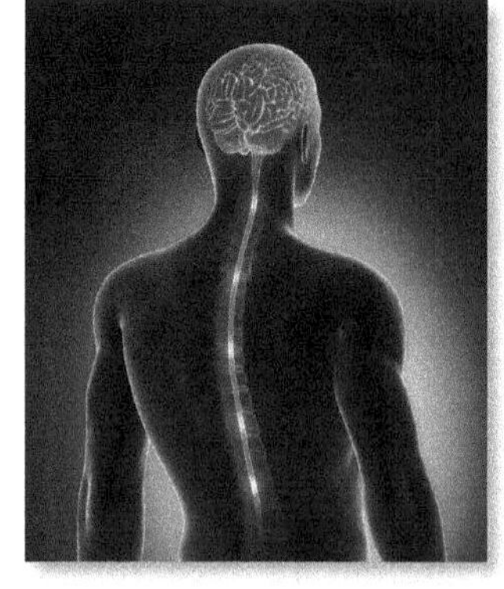

Over the years we have constantly searched for ways to make life better. The drug industry is built on the promise that a pill can make you feel better. There are many diseases and problems that have been treated in this way.

Today we are learning more and more about how drugs affect the body. Almost every day, if you can watch TV, you will find a drug or a surgical procedure that is the target of a new lawsuit. This is because the effects and side effects of drugs on the body can and do vary, and in some cases the outcome is worse than the disease! (http://www.drugwatch.com/drug-lawsuits.php)

When you use medicine alone to treat a disease, you will suffer on some level from the effects the drug causes in your body! If you take a pill to rid yourself of the pain signals your body is sending, you may interfere with a critical process of healing that needs to take place. Pain and other symptoms are just your body's way of getting your attention!

Because everything is connected, you can't treat your body like a machine with replaceable parts!

Because everything is connected, you can't treat your body like a machine with replaceable parts! No matter how much technology advances, science simply cannot replace the normal, smooth processes your body performs each minute of every day.

When we try to replace a part in your body with a new engineered part or support your body with a drug, we interfere with other body processes and this always causes problems. Even something as simple as aspirin will block the ability of the blood to clot normally, so people who have problems with ulcers or bleed easily can't take this drug for pain!

Here is a really simple thing for you to consider…your car, if you own one, is completely replaceable. If you had to, you could go out and get a brand new car even better than the one you drive today! Your body is different. You can't get a new one at any dealer I know of, and getting replacement parts is nearly impossible, even with all of the technology currently available.

You put gas in your car to make the car run. You put food in your mouth to make your body run. But, most of us will choose the best-tasting food instead of choosing the food that is the best for our body! You would never put sugar in your gas tank if you want your car to run, but many people use sugar in every meal, which may lead to diabetes and other diseases as we age! One of the biggest problems we see in health care today is people who want a miracle cure for a disease that is totally preventable with regular, daily attention.

Research done at The Barrow Institute reveals the most important factor in your outcome is where you focus your attention! If you focus on failure, or some way around what you know will cause a successful outcome, you will not get what you want from your efforts! (http://www.barrowneuro.org)

Most of us can focus only on four things at one time. This is why we lose focus and violate the health principles we know will work. We simply take our eye off of the goals we set and when this happens, we cheat ourselves in that momentary lapse!

The real problem with the American way of life is it has taught us from a very young age that we can do anything we want at any moment. This may be fine when applied to some areas of life, but when it is used as a standard for health, the results are usually disastrous!

I had a patient who was a lovely woman. She had a great family, wonderful husband who loved her, great children, and the usual handful of troubles we all have in life. The one thing she did consistently wrong when it came to her life was she ate the most horrible diet.

As a result,, over the years she gained a lot of weight. She was so affected by her diet (which was mainly fast food…think golden arches) that her body literally shut down. Over the years, her habit of drinking diet soda (2, 4, 6 & 10) gave her a tumor in her brain. Then her entire body began to shut down and her doctors could not help her any more. She was in the hospital on a liquid diet, and she was still gaining weight after several days! (http://www.diet.com/g/liquid-diets)

This is an example of what happened to one person. We all have vital body processes that take place on a moment-to-moment basis. If we do one thing wrong, we could suffer a fatal result!

I constantly tell people the same little story in my practice. Your body is a temple, a treasure, a gift, a shrine, and a Maserati (or insert your dream car) all rolled into one! If you take care of it every day, it will last you a lifetime. If you don't, you will suffer as it breaks down!

New research confirms the fact that we are all born with a certain set of genetic, or inborn, factors that we must live with throughout our lives. What it also confirms is that ***you can affect the way every gene expresses itself!*** This means that there are cases where a disease runs in a family, but it does not express itself in one or more members of the family! Even if you get a genetic trait from your bloodline, you can still alter the way the trait affects your life. (http://www.hsph.harvard.edu/obesity-prevention-source/obesity-causes/genes-and-obesity)

So, even if you have some horrible disease from birth, you can prevent the worst parts of the disease (a slow, painful death would be my worst) by doing the best you can to keep your body working like the temple it is! Keep this one thought in mind, and you will see that health is a reward for constant effort on your part! Medicine and all of its parts is here to help you achieve your health goals, not to give them to you and your family!

If you and your family use medical care to help you improve your health, and to intervene when your body can't overcome a disease, you will have a better, more enjoyable life! Currently, there is an argument being pushed by politicians that medical care is a right. As doctors, we are on the other side of this argument for one reason… if medical care is a right, then how are we to treat those who do not value their health?

If everything is connected, and everything you do affects your health, where does our responsibility as doctors end if healthcare is a right? The problem with this position is it creates an endless stream of problems for health care workers and gives the patient less and less control and responsibility. If we will not care for ourselves, we cannot push the end result onto someone else.

If you don't take care of your body, you suffer in the end. Begin by making small, meaningful changes in things you can control. Eat better food, drink better drinks (water!), and exercise!

Don't do these things because you like them, do them because you want the steady, life-enhancing benefits they are guaranteed to give you! You will notice that you have more energy, a better attitude (because being in pain sucks rocks), and a longer, fuller life!

Don't try to make huge changes all at the same time. When I tried for years to get rid of sugar in my diet, I failed miserably! Then I decided that I needed to lose 20 pounds. I tried every type of diet known to man, Atkins, South Beach, you name it, I did it. They all worked. But after I quit the diet, the weight came back, plus 5 or 10 pounds! I convinced myself that I was just more muscular (than the average bear).

Then, at 52, I got serious. My wife had just done a diet that we were using in our office and she lost 15 pounds and kept it off. Now it was my turn! In 23 days I lost 20 pounds! No sugar and no more cravings for sugar. In fact, after this diet (we'll tell you more about it later), I felt really horrible whenever I ate sugar and I don't like it that much anymore! What a great result!

The reason I told you that story is to impress on you the ***fact*** that I, too, have struggles! Every day I make choices, and my choices sometimes get the better of me. I hated myself for not being able to get the sugar out of my diet. I felt weak and stupid, but eventually I found a way to do it! Here is the point...you can do it, too! Whatever the obstacle, ***you are still in control of you!*** Get busy and never stop trying to get better!

Look at the story I just told you and you'll see a truth that repeats itself over and over...even those in health care who know better make excuses at times! You can still go into a hospital (even a cancer center) where they ***know smoking causes disease and death*** and find people outside smoking during a break! Some of these people may even work directly with the patients who are there for cancer treatment!

So, now that you know that everything you do has a direct impact on your health and your life, let's give you the power to make the changes you want! Let's work together without all of the politics and opinions that cloud the issue of responsibility and put you in control. Begin by doing ***one thing***, and repeat this habit until you get the health and the life you deserve!

You will be happier, more productive, have more energy, have more money (because you won't be spending the money in the clinic or the hospital), and you will enjoy your life much more than before! ***What an outcome!***

I could write an entire book on this one topic, but there is a lot of other information that you need to help you get better and stay better. With that in mind, keep this connection of all systems in mind as we go on.

Patients often ask me why they have a specific problem. The one thing I can't do is break a person apart and fix one thing. No doctor or surgeon can! If they cut one part of you, you still get cut!

The same thing applies to any type of drug therapy. When you take a drug, if you take it by mouth, it has to go through your stomach and the intestines. This means the drug gets into the blood, and then it gets into the cells in every part of the body. So, that innocent little aspirin or Tylenol you took for pain also went to your heart, liver, kidneys, and to almost every cell in your body! (http://www.projectknow.com/research/effects-of-drug-abuse/)

I remember when I was young and I felt I could do anything. There was a time when I played every sport imaginable and had a great time doing it. Now I remember all of the injuries and the insults I inflicted on my body and mind, proving I was an athlete.

As I age, I look around at people who are the same age or maybe a bit younger. They look a bit worse for the wear than I do. So, most people have suffered the effects of aging worse than I have.

If you will simply avoid doing things that will hurt you, you will have a better life!

What I have done is learn. I have learned what helps me, and I know what will hurt me. I try my best not to do anything that hurts me. My advice to you is the same. If you will simply avoid doing things that will hurt you, you will have a better life!

But, what if you have a job that ***requires you to lift all day?*** Unfortunately, there are people who have very stressful (physically or mentally stressful) jobs. If you are one of those people, do the very best you can to make sure you are ready for work and able to endure the stress before it happens.

There are many studies that show that preparing for an event or stress will limit the damage you get from the stress. So, the rule here again, is to be prepared! ***(http://www.mindtools.com/selfconf.html)***

Remember that everything you do to your body or your mind will have an effect. These effects can sometimes cause your entire life to be altered as a result of the effect. I want each and every person who reads this book to understand that last sentence…everything you do or think has an impact!

The power of that statement means you have a choice…choose wrong and the impact/effect will be bad; choose right and the impact will be good. It's really that simple. To make sure you get the effect you want, think about what you want out of life and make sure you do as many good/right things to help yourself to that goal as you can!

If you are one of those souls who lives a tortured life, who cannot help themselves and cannot make good choices in life, understand that as much as I care about you and your problem, I cannot overcome your right to choose.

Unfortunately, those in our society who lack the motivation or the self-control to do better do exist. For these people, the only choice is to get help. If they get control of their lives, they can do better. If they can't, they will live and suffer as a result of poor choices until they eventually die. My point here is to make you understand that the choices we make add up as we grow old. This is why we see so many older people who suffer daily as a result of poor health choices they made earlier in life.

You can control every aspect of life if you want to. All you need to do is make the decision to change and make sure you are committed to the change with your whole heart and mind! Your health is really up to you!

Action Plan for Improved Health

1. Write down your health goals for as long as you think you can commit to the plan. If you can only realistically keep these promises for a day, start with just one day and build on that plan!
2. Look at your bad habits and do the research for what this habit will do to your health if you continue it for the rest of your life. Then see if you can commit to change that one thing for a period of time.
3. Commit to a change as a part of your ***lifestyle***, don't exchange habits or replace a lifestyle change with something that has no reward, or worse, feels like you are being penalized!
4. Make sure others in your life understand and support your new goals. If you need one, get a buddy who will cheer you on, if needed, and who will hold you accountable if you slip up.
5. If you fall back into a bad habit (we all DO), make sure you realize that a slip is only one moment of weakness and not a massive life failure. Start over and begin again with day one, then recommit to success!

4

The Two Most Important Things You *Can* Control

When I was training for my Nurse Practitioner degree, we had a course which dealt exclusively with things you, the patient, can control. In the book, they called these things ***modifiable disease risk factors***. These are things you can do to make sure you don't get sick from things you may do.

The wisdom of these modifiable risks is, if you don't lose control of these things, you will be healthier. It doesn't guarantee you an exceptional level of health; it means you may prevent a life-ending disease from causing you pain or death.

The two most preventable risk factors are smoking and excess weight (obesity). The reasons for the importance of these two factors should be pretty easy for most people to understand.

Smoking

Smoking is a direct cause, or can be linked as a cause, in so many diseases that there is no actual count of the number! We know (for a fact) that smoking will eventually kill you, even if you only smoke a little every day. We also know that if you smoke while you are pregnant, smoking will affect your unborn child, and results in lower birth-weights and less healthy babies. (http://www.cdc.gov/tobacco/data_statistics/fact_sheets/health_effects/effects_cig_smoking/)

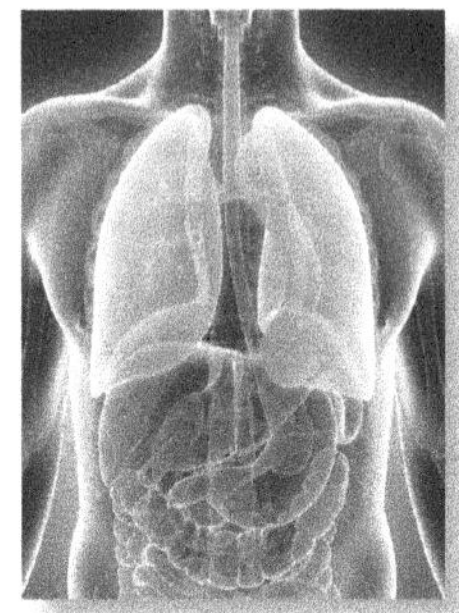

Smoking will damage your lungs, one of the most important organs in your body. Simply put, if you can't breathe, you won't live very long! If you smoke, not only do you damage your lungs, but you also cause damage to other tissues that need oxygen (which is ***all of them***).

Over the course of your life, you will lose 10 years of your life if you smoke without quitting. When you quit, your body will heal, but it will never be as good as it was before you began smoking. (http://www.newscientist.com/article/dn6054-smoking-wipes-10-years-off-a-life.html)

We had a patient who had smoked for many years. She was loved by her family and her husband. As she got older, her health began to decline rapidly! It was almost scary how fast she lost her health and her ability to function.

She developed a condition called chronic obstructive pulmonary disease (COPD). This condition robbed her of her ability to even walk without being hooked up to a portable oxygen tank. Her health got worse day by day until she died. The point of this story is, other than smoking, this lady was doing nothing else wrong! (http://www.ncbi.nlm.nih.gov/pubmedhealth/PMH0001153/)

Smoking damages your body in a lot of really bad ways. So let's look at a few of the first things you should consider before you light up. We know, for sure, that smoking any type of tobacco, dipping or chewing, will cause cancer (all types of cancer).

Cancer is a terrible disease on any level. What happens in cancer is the cells of the tumor don't die like other cells in our body do. The result is an uncontrolled growth of cells that are not like the other cells in your body.

Unfortunately, the cancer cells can and do take over blood supply, which will affect the nutrition to the other cells in the body. The result is the cancer grows and overtakes the body, and the person eventually dies!

Smoking also causes other problems. Outside of the obvious bad breath, you will damage any tissue in your body that gets exposed to the smoke or tobacco. The damage begins in your mouth. You damage your teeth, which get stained at first, and then with continued tobacco use, begin to erode and change in other horrible ways.

When I was young I went to the dentist to get my wisdom teeth pulled. In the other room was a young man who was having a terrible time. He was moaning so loudly from his pain that it was unnerving. The dentist showed me his x-rays which revealed such bad erosion of his teeth that his lower jaw was literally eaten up from decay. This was all caused from dipping tobacco!

Now consider the damage tobacco does to the esophagus and your bronchial tree (the tubes that go to your stomach and lungs). If tobacco can damage and ruin your teeth, it will ***destroy*** the soft tissues and organs in your body!

If tobacco can damage and ruin your teeth, it will destroy the soft tissues and organs in your body!

There are many different ways to quit smoking after you start. I tell all of my patients (especially the young ones) that the best way to avoid the problems caused by smoking is to never start in the first place. The nicotine in tobacco actually causes addiction by exciting the nerve centers in your brain that cause addiction to heroin. These are very powerful nerve endings, which is why it is so hard to quit for most people who try. (http://www.ncbi.nlm.nih.gov/pmc/articles/PMC3025154/)

However, if you already smoke, you don't need that piece of sage advice! You need strategies to quit.

Here are some ways you may consider when you decide to stop! First, you must make the decision to quit. Whatever reason you choose, make sure it is vitally important to you and failing to make the goal of quitting will cause you pain! Your decision to quit should be documented and the date you plan to begin should be written down. Give yourself specific goals and rewards for completion. (http://quitsmoking.about.com/od/preparetoquit/u/quitting.htm)

Look into all of the ways you can get help and pick a way that ***feels right to you***.

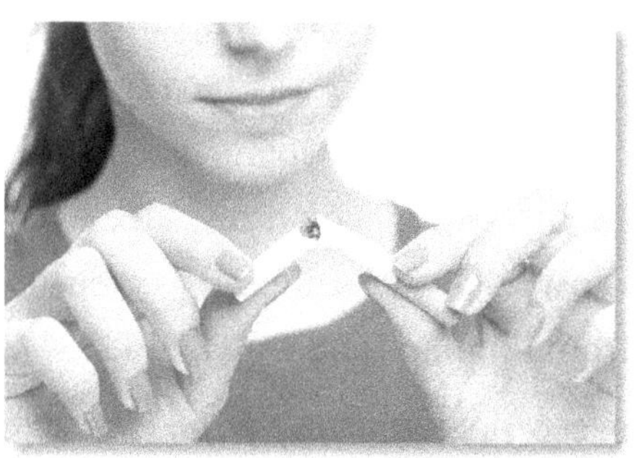

Cold turkey - this is the simplest and direct approach. You just stop without any help on a day you choose and you never light up again!

Medical assistance - several drugs work to help curb the nicotine addiction and cravings. Nicotine replacement therapy (NRT) uses patches, gum, spray, lozenges, or an inhaler to replace the nicotine and help you smoke less while you quit.

Chantix and Zyban are drugs that work by decreasing the cravings and urges to smoke caused by nicotine. Chantix can be used while you smoke, and Zyban can be used with NRT. The big thing to understand is, all drugs have side effects. Chantix and Zyban both have side effects that you need to be aware of before you begin using them. (http://www.cdc.gov/tobacco/campaign/tips/quit-smoking/guide/explore-medications.html)

Acupuncture - I have seen ads and have been in clinics where the doctor or practitioner claimed he/she was able to get rid of smoking addiction with acupuncture treatment.

Some of the clinics had cigarette packages stacked literally floor to ceiling. The doctors proudly told me that each pack was the last pack a particular patient had smoked before he treated them. I have used several different formulae on several different patients, but I have never been able to reproduce this claimed level of success.

In fact, I was asked to do acupuncture by a major corporation for its employees and I declined due to this fact! Later, I was told by the nurse that the program had been implemented (by an acupuncture school), and only one person had been able to quit for more than six months.

There may be someone out there who is an acupuncture genius with high levels of success, but until I see the results, I'll just say I am skeptical if this method works to stop addiction or smoking. Ask for references from actual people who were successfully treated for smoking.

If the doctor can provide enough good, quality references, and you want to try this method, go ahead! The real truth is, for almost every other problem acupuncture has value and is very safe. (http://www.doctoroz.com/blog/jamie-starkey-lac/acupuncture-can-help-you-kick-habit)

Hypnosis - the doctor or therapist will put you into a trance or altered state and give you suggestions to help decrease your cravings for smoking and nicotine. If you are able to be hypnotized, this may work for you. Again, please get references of people the therapist has helped and who have been smoke-free for long enough to make them well!

Will power - no matter which method you choose, your will to quit is the one thing that will have the greatest impact and increase your odds of quitting for good. You, and you alone, are the one factor in the whole equation that can tip the odds in favor of quitting or failing! All of the research proves those who make a firm and unyielding decision to quit, and are committed to success, are those who stop smoking and never smoke again!

Your brain and your will are the most important factors, and will be the reasons you quit for good. Here are other tips that may help you quit. (http://quitsmoking.about.com/od/howtoquitsmoking/a/quit_smoking.htm)

Action Plan to Stop Smoking

1. When you make the decision to stop smoking it is a cause for celebration, but don't celebrate in a way that may cause you to smoke! Remember that you have triggers that may cause you to crave a cigarette. Drinking and being around others who smoke will make it harder for you.
2. Dopamine is the hormone you secrete when you smoke a cigarette. This substance is the core of your addiction (as well as nicotine). To get past your addiction, you must stay focused and stay in charge! Write down your commitment to quit and ask a coach or a buddy to help you in times when you feel the urge to smoke again. (http://bigthink.com/going-mental/your-brain-on-drugs-dopamine-and-addiction)
3. If you can't quit cold-turkey, reduce the number of cigarettes you smoke each day, use NRT or medications to help curb your urges until you can comfortably stop smoking. Try putting your cigarettes in a place that is out of your way so you don't have easy access to a smoke when you get cravings.
4. If you respond better to positive feedback, reward yourself for progress. If negative feedback helps, write a list of all the costs and problems associated with smoking and emphasize the lifetime cost of the cigarettes. Then add in the potential diseases you may develop and look up the cost of these diseases. Remember, you may have more than one disease from smoking and you may have more costs if you look at the physical damage smoking does to your body and possessions!
5. Track your progress daily and keep after your goal of being smoke-free! Even if it takes you ten years to stop smoking, your

body will heal. Never, ever, ever give up! (http://www.becomeanex.org/create-profile.php#)

Obesity - being overweight

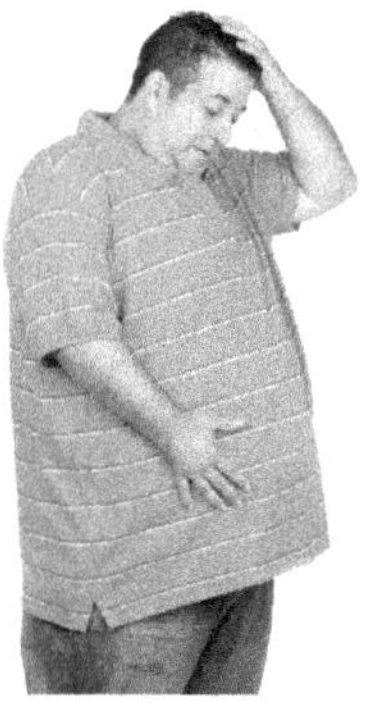

Being overweight is a dangerous way to live. Over the years, we have treated many people in our office who were suffering the effects of carrying too much weight on their joints for too many years. Over the course of their lives they began to notice joint pain, body aches, and a severe loss of energy and an inability to work or play like they used to.

Obesity is defined as having a Body Mass Index (BMI) of 30 or over. You get your BMI by dividing your weight (in kilograms) by your height (in meters). (http://www.obesityaction.org/understanding-obesity/obesity)

There are over 44 different diseases that are related to being overweight! The most commonly known conditions related to obesity are high blood pressure, high cholesterol, and diabetes. Other conditions are not so well known, like cancer! (http://www.cdc.gov/healthyweight/effects/)

We know a lot about how to lose weight! But just like smoking, weight problems are unique to each person. If you are overweight and need to lose more than just a few pounds, the task can become overwhelming. The biggest obstacle you must overcome is the daily barrage of temptation. Make up your mind to ignore these problems and you will succeed!

We had a patient who was obese. She needed to lose at least half of her total body weight just to be considered overweight by medical standards! We talked about her problem and she told me she didn't like exercise because she didn't like to sweat.

She began to eat less at each meal and all she did for exercise was walk in the shallow end of the community pool. No sweating, and the result after just three months was a loss of over 40 pounds! This proves that with just a little bit of help, you can reach any goal you are committed to!

If your problem is a love of food, remember that you are in control! Don't allow anything without a brain to control you in any way! The other thing you must understand is how your weight can get out of control.

After looking all over, and doing research on almost every diet, I found out what may be the most important bit of information related to weight. If you eat just 10 calories per day more than you burn, you will gain on average almost ten pounds per year!

The big problem is, ten calories per day is ***very easy*** to eat! It is literally one Tic Tac mint per day…almost nothing, when you think about it. So we must all accept this one truth. If you don't constantly stay in control of what and how much you eat, your weight will get out of control. (http://pediatrics.about.com/od/obesity/a/06_calpound_fat.htm)

One of the most asked questions we get regarding weight is, "How can I lose the weight?" What people really want is to know how to lose the weight *without suffering*. If you are like me and you love bread and sweets, it's impossible to lose weight without sacrifice.

I thought for years that I had a real addiction to sugar. Then, after doing some research for this book, I found out that I was also sensitive to gluten.

Gluten is in a lot of foods that we eat. It is used as a binder (something that makes food stick together) in a ton of recipes and store-bought food. My problem was I had bad headaches that would turn into migraines if I didn't get the right amount of sleep each day.

As you may guess, I was having these headaches more often than I care to admit. The gluten in my food was also keeping me from losing weight. These two issues got me to finally try gluten-free eating for three weeks.

The results were nothing short of amazing! I lost weight, felt better, and had almost no headaches (even with little sleep) after just three weeks. I have been able to stay mainly gluten-free for months now, and the benefits keep coming!

I sacrificed my love of bread because I knew that I couldn't go on living with the headaches and weight gain caused by gluten sensitivity. There are times when I wish I could eat like I used to...but then I remember those headaches.

As much as I'd love a piece of warm, out-of-the-oven bread or some cake, I really don't want those headaches! I have made the choice to give up gluten, even though I still crave it.

You, too, must let go of those things that are not really that good for you, but taste wonderful. I tell my patients that it's fairly easy to lose weight if you follow some simple guidelines.

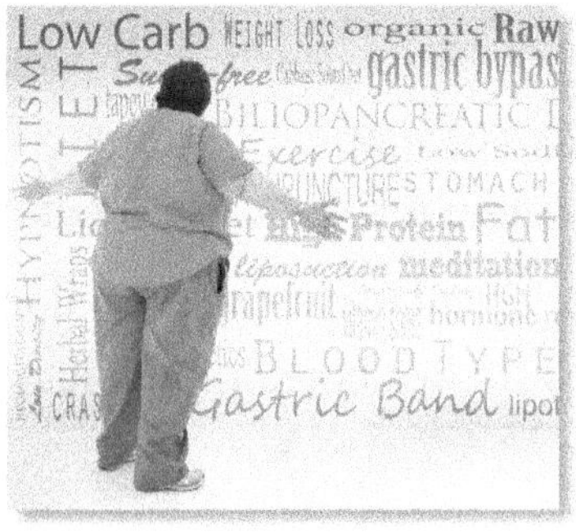

Action Plan for Weight Loss

1. Don't eat sugar, or anything that converts to sugar quickly in your mouth. This includes bread and empty calorie starches (rice, pasta, white potatoes, chips and crackers).
2. Don't starve yourself. When most people diet, they try and fail because they eat too little food. Eat six small meals per day (including regular snacks of nuts and non-tropical fruit). You should eat twice as many vegetable servings as protein, and your protein portions should be smaller than the palm of your hand.
3. Drink water, water, water! No sugar drinks or sodas. We recommend no diet sodas either, but if you must drink soda, drink no-sugar soda. If you use sugar substitutes, we recommend Stevia.
4. Commit to your new lifestyle and recognize that small changes will result in big changes in the future. You can change your body just by changing your mind and by being consistent.
5. Exercise is important, but only do exercise that you will repeat! You only need about 30 minutes per day and it will change you forever! Find something you like (walking, swimming, etc.), then add or change the exercise so your body doesn't stagnate. Use the Internet for help! (http://www.webmd.com/fitness-exercise/ss/slideshow-7-most-effective-exercises)

5

Colds, Flu, Allergies and Other Breathing Problems

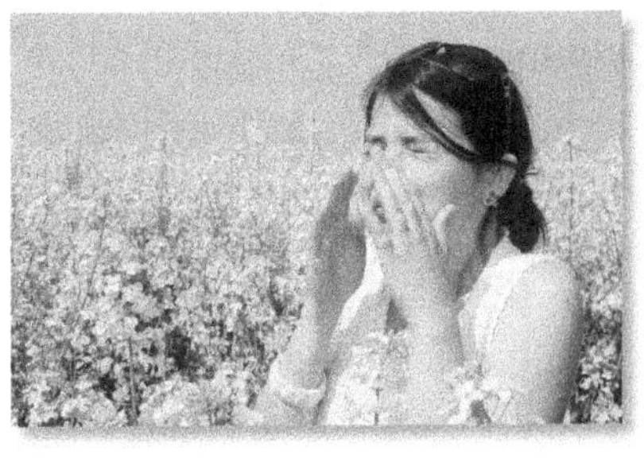

Most people have had a cold or the flu at one time or another in their life. During the "cold and flu season," doctors' offices and hospitals see an overall increase in the number of patients who want to be seen, and there are also more people who are very ill and require hospitalization.

Every year, when this season approaches, people ask me the same question… "Doctor, why do I get sick from this year after year?"

… the main reason we are healthier in the spring and summer is we go outside!

The truth about cold and flu season is it really exists all year long! Colds and flu are caused mainly by viruses that exist in our bodies in our mouths, and the tissues of our nose, throat and lungs. So why do we get sick in the winter and not in the summer? Simply put, the main reason we are healthier in the spring and summer is we go outside!

When we are outside, we aren't exposed to the concentration of bugs that others around us breathe into the air. We get a small dose from them if we are in the vicinity, but not as much as we get when we are inside and someone who is sick sneezes or coughs!

But what really keeps you and me healthy is our immune system. It is this system that fights off any type of disease or illness and makes sure you survive. If your immunity is high, you have a powerful resistance to any disease, but when your immunity is low, you get sick more easily.

Unfortunately for most of us, as we age we get sick more frequently because of the natural decline of our body systems and the combined effects of our lifestyle. This means that it may take less exposure to germs for us to get sick year after year!

So, how do the medical doctors fix this? And what are the options that you can use to help yourself? Let's take a look at the options for health side by side.

When you get the flu

The Medical Approach

Tamiflu - a drug that helps your body fight off the flu after you get it. You must take it (Tamiflu) within two days of getting the flu or it won't work!

Side effects from using Tamiflu include: nausea, vomiting, diarrhea, nosebleeds, dizziness, headaches, and other things that may be nastier (if you are allergic to the medicine that fights the flu).

How it works: Tamiflu is made in a controlled way to work by binding or blocking the receptor sites on the flu virus that let the virus penetrate your cell walls. When this happens, the virus makes copies of itself and you get sick. By blocking this action, Tamiflu stops the virus from making copies of itself, and this is how the drug works! (http://www.edinformatics.com/interactive_molecules/tamiflu.htm)

Antibiotics - There are times when antibiotics work for an illness, but when you get the flu, this is one of the times when the drug will not work! Antibiotics work on bacterial diseases; the flu is caused by a virus, so no antibiotic will work when you have the flu. At times, a doctor will give an antibiotic to a patient who has more than one cause of illness, for instance, when a patient has a bacterial infection or pneumonia and the flu.

How it works: Antibiotics work by selectively killing bacteria or by slowing the growth of bacteria in your body so your body can heal itself.

The Flu Vaccine - There are always a lot of questions about the vaccine. As a medical professional, I *always* tell my patients that they should get vaccinated. Many of the vaccines we have today prevent the diseases that have killed millions.

That said, please do your own research and look specifically at the Centers for Disease Control website for the *most current information!* There was an article in Time Magazine that stated, "Influenza is a notoriously wily virus and known to mutate quickly and effectively to evade confrontation with immune defenses generated by a vaccine." (www.cdc.gov/flu/)

What *Time* said in plain English is every vaccine for the flu gives the person taking it a helping hand. However, the ones we produce are hardly ever a perfect match for the actual virus that makes people sick. You may get some benefit from the current vaccine, but don't count on the vaccine to keep you from getting the current strain of flu! (http://www.webmd.com/vaccines/how-effective-is-flu-vaccine)

Some things that are always repeated each flu season are:

1. "If I get the vaccine, it contains some parts of the actual flu virus, so it may make me sick." Actually, the ***nasal vaccine*** called "Flu-mist" is the only vaccine with parts of the virus in the vaccine. Other types do not contain parts of the actual virus that give a person the flu! What you may get is a sore spot where the vaccine is injected, but the injection is small (usually only 1/2 of one cc), so it doesn't even hurt that much if done properly!
2. "All vaccines have that mercury stuff, and it's really bad and can make you sicker than the flu!" Again, that mercury stuff (called Thimerosal), is not in many of the vaccines. You can simply ask for a Thimerosal-free vaccine to avoid this concern.
3. "I get the vaccine, so I won't get sick!" This is not really true, either. There will always be a certain percentage of people who get the vaccine at the right time, but still get sick from the current strain of flu. You get the flu because your immune system is not strong enough to prevent you from getting sick. If your immune system is compromised or weak, you may get the flu ***in spite of the fact that you got vaccinated!***

All of the current research is out there for you to find. As usual, the Internet has an opinion for everyone and everybody! Just be sure you get more than one educated opinion before you make up your mind what path you take!

The Natural Approach

Avoiding the flu is really about maintaining your body's natural defenses. You can avoid the flu by keeping your immune system strong. This is done on a daily basis by eating right, getting exercise during the flu months to keep your body strong, and by doing simple things like washing your hands and not drinking after people who may be sick!

These things can make your chances of getting sick less, but may not prevent an episode of the flu. We also recommend using zinc (in a nasal spray or lozenge) in combination with Vitamin C with rose hips. (http://a-renewedhealth.com/rose_hips)

There is another product called Emergen-C which is a natural mix of vitamins (high dose of Vitamin C and others) and minerals which may help your immune system fight off a cold or the flu if used before you get really sick. You need to be careful in some cases when you take high doses of vitamins (vitamins A, D, E, and K can build up and cause vitamin poisoning/toxicity). (http://www.emergenc.com/)

There are some people who like to use a product called Colloidal Silver. I have personally used this for other types of problems and some studies do show silver can get into the outer protective membrane of bacteria and viruses. ***However***, there are recorded instances where people overused the silver solution and turned their skin ***BLUE!*** (http://www.rsc.org/chemistryworld/2012/11/chemistry-blue-man-argyria-colloidal-silver)

So, the rule on all remedies is simple… NEVER use more than the recommended amount for any reason! Even the gentlest product can cause problems when used too much or for the wrong reasons! There is a load of other products out there that claim to be effective when the cold and flu season hits every year. ***Use your own mind and make the best choices by doing the research!*** If you want the opinion of others who have used a specific product, use Google and ask for "reviews." It's an absolutely fabulous tool!

Even the gentlest product can cause problems when used too much or for the wrong reasons!

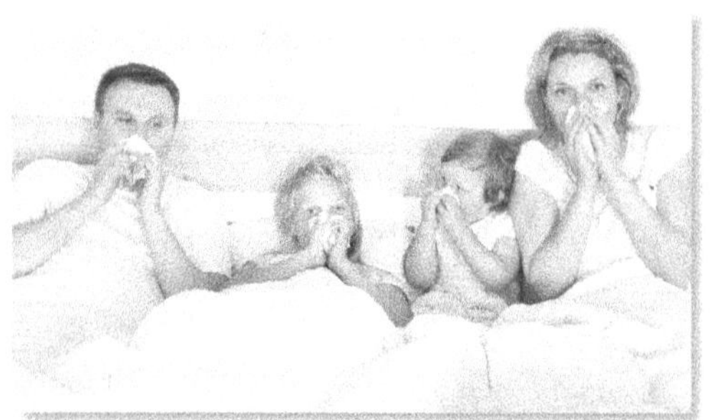

If you use these items, understand what you are doing is helping your body by making it harder for any virus to survive inside of your body by using totally natural methods. If we could get the high quality foods our great-grandparents had when they were growing up, we probably wouldn't need supplements to help us stay well.

However, today, we have what we have, and unless you have the land to farm and grow natural foods without all of the additives and chemicals, you will have to make do with the local grocer. He probably gets his produce and meat from the big corporate farms that make most of the food we can all buy.

What can you do if you get the flu? Unfortunately, the truth is, not much. Because the flu is caused by a virus, you need to let the infection run its course. If you get too sick, it's time to go to the doctor and get some help! You need to make a decision about what you consider to be unacceptable for you or a family member. Here are some simple guidelines for you to consider…

What can you do if you get the flu? Unfortunately, the truth is, not much.

Ages 0-4: At this age, the danger is allowing a fever to get too far out of range and causing other problems. In very young people, this can happen quickly and can be very dangerous. If the child is playing normally and is eating and acting well, a fever of 99° F is not too high.

But if the fever gets over 101°, and the child is not acting, playing or eating like normal, then they need medical attention. One of the most dangerous signals is when a child gets very clingy and won't eat or drink. This can be a sign of a loss of too much fluid, or dehydration, which can lead to serious problems if not remedied quickly.

Many times, if an infant gets a temperature of 100° (100.2° is the real number) rectally, the rule is to go ***immediately to the emergency room at the nearest hospital!*** Babies and small children have very fragile systems that can be damaged for life if they get ill and a fever is allowed to damage the delicate brain cells.

We had a child and his mother in the office with the exact symptoms I described above. This little boy had been sick for two days, but his mother thought he would get better. We had to keep him in the office for two hours while we tried in vain to get him to drink fluid to get his fever down, but after two hours, the trial time was up, and we had to send him to the hospital. He had to have the fluid pushed into his body with an IV (the hospital used a needle and forcibly put fluid into his body through a vein). This was done even though we told the child he may have to go to the hospital and he ***really didn't want to go!***

Ages 4 to adult: During these years, we can handle a bit more. Make sure you don't allow the suffering to go too far, and use the following to speed your healing and make your down time more tolerable. Fever over 103° is a problem and needs medical attention. You can make your symptoms better when your fever is lower than 100° by taking a hot bath. A hot bath can get your temperature up and can help burn off the infection to a small degree.

Make sure you keep water next to the tub while you soak *and drink it* to keep your body hydrated. You also need to make sure you check your temperature regularly to make sure you don't get your body temperature up too high! (http://children.webmd.com/tc/fever-age-4-and-older-topic-overview)

After your bath, try using a washcloth (use an old one) with castor oil drizzled on it. Put the cloth on your body wherever you hurt and cover it with a heating pad on low heat. This has a wonderful effect of decreasing the soreness in the area without causing you to lose more fluid.

Some patients have asked me, "Doctor, if the fever is my body's way of burning off an infection, why is a high fever dangerous?"

The answer to this question is simple. When your fever gets too high, your body may lose the ability to bring it back down to a normal temperature. It's almost like you get a short circuit in the computer program that runs and regulates your body.

If this happens, ***especially if or when it happens to a child***, the situation can go from bad to emergency within minutes. Children are so much more sensitive, and may react badly to a fever, that they have much lower tolerances. You must pay attention to your child, and be ready and willing to take them to the emergency room if you have to! (http://www.mayoclinic.org/diseases-conditions/fever/basics/symptoms/con-20019229)

I recently read a book about a neurosurgeon who almost died. He went to bed with a headache, but because he took a hot bath and the bath made him feel better, he ignored the condition. He woke up the next day and still had a bad headache, but because he was a medical professional, he went in to take another bath so he could go to work. His condition did not get any better! (We were told repeatedly in our medical training that a really bad headache should ***never*** be ignored!)

Don't ever let a sign or a symptom of disease go untreated just because you think someone may judge you!

He wrote that he didn't want to be carted off to the ER and be seen as "one of those nervous patients" when they found nothing to treat but the headache. He wound up in a coma for one week and very nearly died as a result of the infection that was causing his headache! (http://www.ebenalexander.com/books/proof-of-heaven/)

This is an example of what could happen if you ignore your body's warning systems. Don't ever let a sign or a symptom of disease go untreated just because you think someone may judge you! I always tell my patients that I prefer they treat a symptom with respect to avoid a bad outcome from neglect.

When you get a cold

If you get a cold, the thing to remember is a cold is caused by a virus, just like the flu. The difference is, you typically don't get as sick from a cold as you will from the flu. Because your symptoms are milder, people typically walk around for days and weeks with colds and this is how the virus spreads to others. Your cold may be just as dangerous to some people (especially those with lower immunity) and may cause them to become very sick if exposed!

To help yourself and help others, simply do your best to keep the illness to yourself! Stay away from very young and very old people who may have weaker immune systems and who could get very ill from your virus. Keep your mouth and nose covered when you cough or sneeze and keep washing your hands.

In order to lessen the impact of the illness, get a lot of rest. I tell patients they need at least one to two more hours of sleep per day to recover their health when they are sick. Your body is a miraculous, organized, and complex thing, so when you are sick, all of your systems need to be reset.

Your brain is still in control, but like a computer, sometimes the best thing to do is to turn it off! Sleep is your body's way of resetting all of the systems and it is your brain's way of shutting down like a computer that has been shut off.

Eat only good food when you are sick! I see many people who go out and get food that ***tastes good, but isn't good for them***. This can make the sickness last longer! If you owned the most expensive car in the world, would you put sugar in the gas tank if the car was running rough? Of course not! So why eat sugar and other zero-quality foods when you feel bad?

Sugar ***always*** causes swelling and inflammation of the body when you eat it. I have found that if I eliminate sugar, or anything that turns into sugar quickly in the body, I don't get sick as often, and if I do get sick I don't stay sick as long!

The other benefit is that reducing sugar makes all of the other foods I eat taste better! Sugar does provide a quick burst of energy, but the energy provided won't give your body the needed calories to help it heal. I always regret eating sugar when I am ill. The crash I feel after a sugar high makes me feel worse when I am sick.

Action Plan for Colds and Flu

1. Make sure to do all of the things that prevent colds and flu before you get sick. If you are high risk, get vaccinated ***before cold and flu season!***
2. Keep your immune system functioning at its best by exercising and eating right all year long.
3. Use common sense to keep yourself and those who are around you healthy. Wash your hands regularly, eat quality, low-sugar foods, don't share drinks or eat after others, and make sure you keep up your exercise routine!
4. If you get sick, understand your body needs more rest! Sleep is one of the best things you can do to help yourself heal faster! Get plenty of rest and don't rush back to work unless it's absolutely necessary.
5. Make sure and disinfect your toothbrush and go ahead and buy a new one you can use after you are well. Don't sweat the $2.00 for a new toothbrush; it's way better than getting sick again after a cold or flu bout!

Allergies

Allergies are simply a reaction to a substance that becomes an irritant to your system. Many people suffer with allergies. The most common problems associated with allergies are sneezing, breathing problems, and runny nose. If an allergy becomes too severe, the person who suffers with it may have an extreme reaction called anaphylaxis, which is life-threatening. (http://www.nlm.nih.gov/medlineplus/ency/article/000844.htm)

If you know someone who has a severe allergy, the best course of action is to avoid the substance (or allergen) altogether! Even a small amount of an allergen can be too much for a person with an anaphylactic reaction, and the resulting reaction to any exposure could be fatal.

Luckily for most of us, we know when we are extremely sensitive to foods or other things that cause allergies. Most people do not have an anaphylactic reaction to common things, and those who do usually carry an epi-pen (epinephrine) in case of emergency.

Medical Approach

The medical approach to treating allergies is actually a bit weird! Doctors initially will give you antihistamines and decongestants. They will also give you instructions to stay away from the allergens if you can. If these things do not work, then the doctor will refer you to an allergist, who will begin treating you with small amounts of the substances you are allergic to in order to desensitize you to the substance. (http://www.webmd.com/allergies/guide/allergies-treatment-care)

How treatments work

Antihistamines work by drying up the nasal water-works we get when allergies attack. These drugs work directly on the soft tissues in your nose. The tiny particles that float in the air are inhaled, and then they make your sinuses swell. In an attempt to get rid of the allergen, your body turns the water on! It literally tries to wash out your system by flooding the sinuses (with mucus) and washing the particles out.

Decongestants work by getting the fluid out of your sinuses. It will reduce the full or stuffy feeling you may have as a result of an allergy. But you must be careful with all kinds of drugs. This one can be dangerous for people who have high blood pressure!

Nasal Allergy Sprays (steroid and antihistamine combos) work by decreasing the secretions from the glands in your nose and sinuses, but the side effect can be that it causes your nose to be too dry or even to bleed!

Steroid Nasal Sprays work by decreasing the swelling of the nasal tissues, which leads to less mucus or less running of your nose. As with the other sprays, it can lead to a dry or bleeding nose from the effect of the steroids. If this happens, just stop, cut back on your use, or try using saline spray to add moisture to your nose and prevent the bleeding.

Allergy eye drops decrease the watery eyes we sometimes get as a result of being exposed to an allergen. They may be simple saline drops to wash out allergens, or may contain steroids to decrease the swelling and reduce the tears and redness produced by an allergen.

Mast Cell Inhibitors and Leukotriene Inhibitors (Singulair or Astelin) work by stopping the swelling and mucous production that allergies cause. The mast cells inhibitors can be nasal sprays or eye drops and they may have side effects of over-drying the tissues they are working on.

Allergy shots may be used to decrease your sensitivity to the allergen. The doctor gives you a shot with a small amount of the allergen in a liquid to get your body to decrease the reaction to exposure. At first, you will need to get shots frequently, because the amount you get exposed to in each shot is small and the effect seems to wear off quickly.

Over time, the goal is to build up your immunity by repeatedly exposing you to the substance, and the hope is you will tolerate the exposure better with each shot. This approach is what happens to a person who gets stung by bees so many times he doesn't swell or feel the pain of the sting anymore.

Alternative Measures

There are other ways to help yourself without using drugs to slow or stop the effects of allergies in your life.

There are some very impressive studies showing the herb ***butterbur*** works very well for nasal allergies. ***Saline nasal washes*** thin out the mucus and can help wash out any allergens which get into the sinuses. Adding freeze-dried nettles and a tonic made from goldenseal also seems to be effective at reducing or stopping the stuffy or runny nose, and stemming the flow that can make life miserable. (http://www.webmd.com/allergies/features/natural-allergy-relief)

Some have found aid from homeopathic remedies, which are tonics or pills made and used to desensitize the body to the allergic substance. These are made by distilling a substance down in alcohol, and then using the tincture (the distilled or diluted part used to treat a person). There are many people who find these remedies to be helpful, but there are others who are convinced the effects are simply from a placebo effect.

Neuro-Linguistic Programming (NLP) is another tool that has been used to help with allergies with no side effect. The premise of this technique is that the person who suffers from an allergy is simply experiencing the effect of a remembered reaction to a stress which, in effect, is what ***causes the allergic reaction to manifest.*** NLP has made a study of the effects of removing this remembered effect and, in many recorded cases, the allergic symptom was successfully removed. (http://www.nlpu.com/Patterns/pattern9.htm)

Breathing Problems

Breathing problems are very dangerous! In school they told us over and over again, the first rule of medical evaluation was A, B, C…airway, breathing and circulation. If you lose the ability to breathe, you cannot survive. We must always remember that, in the category of most important things to maintain, airway and breathing are number one and two!

If you lose the ability to breathe, you cannot survive.

There are several different kinds of breathing problems. We will discuss the most common types and examine the different types of care you can use to help or prevent these problems.

Sinusitis

This is simply a problem with the lining tissues of your nose and the mucus glands (sinuses) in your face. Your skull has bones in the front that have holes in it. These holes are lined with tissue that warms the air you breathe in through your nose and grab particles that could cause problems if they got into your lungs. The sticky fluid produced in your nose is part of this system.

When you get something in your nose that irritates you, your sinuses produce more fluid to try to wash the irritating particle out. This fluid can build up and cause pressure to build, which can cause headaches and may result in a sinus or respiratory infection if allowed to progress. Almost everyone has had a day where they wake up with a sore throat. This may be caused by sinuses that drain into your throat while you sleep at night.

The big problem with nighttime drainage is it could cause an infection of the upper airway (upper respiratory infection or URI). This could cause or lead to pneumonia, which is a very serious problem and needs to be treated medically. (http://www.mayoclinic.com/health/pneumonia/DS00135/DSECTION=treatments-and-drugs).

Sinus infections occur when you get an infection in the mucus glands inside of your face. The pressure can be so painful that it makes you want to go to bed. The big problem with an infection is it is very hard for you to get rid of without using medication to dry up your sinuses or an antibiotic to help your body overcome the infection.

You will notice your mucus has color (usually yellow or green), and you may have a fever with the infection. Having the green or yellow color means your body is doing its best to fight off the infection! You need to be careful that your body does not get overwhelmed with the fluid produced from your sinuses, as this could lead to pneumonia.

If your sinus problem is long-standing, your doctor may do a test called a sinus computed tomography (CT) or an MRI to see if other problems exist that are making you sick over time. A CT uses x-rays and a computer to take images of the area which give details that cannot be seen on a normal x-ray.

The main treatments for sinus problems have already been discussed. If you have a sinus infection, you will likely have a fever and you will more than likely get antibiotics to help shift your immune system into high gear. You may help yourself by avoiding anything that makes your sinuses stuffy or runny. It may also help to wash your sinuses out with saline or a neti pot. (http://www.webmd.com/allergies/sinus-pain-pressure-11/neti-pots)

Asthma

Asthma happens when a person gets exposed to something that causes the upper airways to swell. This swelling causes the glands in the tissues to produce mucus, which causes coughing and leads to shortness of breath. As the person tries to get air into the lungs, they will often use the muscles in the neck to try to breathe. This "recruiting" of other muscles in order to breathe is typical of a person in distress.

Medical Approach

The medical approach to the treatment of asthma is to avoid the "triggers" that cause asthma, and to treat the symptoms of the attack, bringing the person back to normal, easy breathing. The "real goal" of any breathing problem we treat in medicine is to help the person with the problem live as normally as they can.

This means we should educate the person about the things that he/she can do to make the problem better, and things they shouldn't do (things that will cause the symptoms).

The key to treatment of asthma is early action! If you act quickly, your symptoms will not be as bad. This means you can get back to your life and do the things you love to do without gasping for a breath.

The first line of attack for asthma treatment is usually ***steroids***. There are quick-acting inhalers for emergencies and there are other drugs that are taken to prevent asthma symptoms from starting. The quick-acting drugs are short-acting beta agonists (albuterol - ProAir

HFA, Ventolin HFA, and levalbuterol/Xopenex, or pirbuterol/Max-Air), and Ipatroprium bromide (Atrovent inhaler). (http://www.webmd.com/asthma/guide/asthma-control-with-anti-inflammatory-drugs)

How steroids work

Steroids work by reducing the swelling and the mucus production in the lung tissues which opens the airway and helps you breathe better. As these drugs work, the soft tissues actually decrease in size, which slows or stops the production of more mucus and this helps you breathe more easily. This also may decrease your sensitivity to allergens or things that irritate the tissues of your lungs and cause the breathing problem.

The big thing to remember about steroid drugs is they don't relieve asthma symptoms during an attack!

The big thing to remember about steroid drugs is they don't relieve asthma symptoms during an attack! These drugs are best when used to prevent asthma and need to be taken on a schedule (daily) to work properly.

These drugs are usually inhaled through an inhaler or a metered dose device that basically crushes a pill or blasts a spray into your mouth. You should take a deep breath (if possible), exhale completely, and then put the inhaler in your mouth, inhale, and spray the dose, trying to get the dose as far into your lungs as you can. You are also supposed to try to hold your breath after the dose…but, if you are having an attack, do your best and make sure you know when to get help!

Remember, you must rinse your mouth out with water after you take each dose. This must be done to prevent yeast infections in your mouth that sometimes occur as a side effect of these drugs. Also, these are not the same steroids that body-builders use to get muscle. You will not get ripped muscles from your inhaler, but if you have exercise-induced asthma, you need to take it before you exercise! (http://www.mayoclinic.com/health/exercise-induced-asthma/DS01040/DSECTION=treatments-and-drugs)

Leukotriene modifiers do basically the same thing as steroids, but they work in different ways. These drugs may work for up to 24 hours and suppress the effects of leukotrienes. These chemicals, which cause inflammation and constriction of the muscles in your airway, are in your body and may make an asthma attack worse. (http://www.webmd.com/asthma/guide/asthma-control-with-anti-inflammatory-drugs?page=2)

Mast cell stabilizers are drugs that reduce swelling in the bronchial tubes which lead to your lungs. They help by reducing the tightening of the muscles in the airways, which will make it easier for you to breathe. Unfortunately, these drugs do not work quickly. They must be taken over weeks and sometimes for months, before they decrease asthma.

This is the reason they are in the class called long-term controller medicines. They must be taken daily, regardless of whether or not you are having symptoms and they take a bit of time to work, so you have to keep taking them to get relief. These medicines also need to be monitored over time, so you'll also need to work with your doctor to make sure you don't overuse the medicines and cause dangerous side effects.

One thing you must remember about these medicines is...***they don't work for an asthmatic attack***! If you are having an asthmatic episode, you can't breathe NOW. Taking your mast cell stabilizer (Cromolyn Sodium and Tilade are examples) during the attack simply won't help when you can't breathe. If you are having an attack, you need to take the fast-acting emergency drugs mentioned above! (http://www.mayoclinic.com/health/drug-information/DR601675)

Side effects

The side effects of these drugs are skin rashes, coughing, irritation of your throat, some psychological problems (hallucinations, agitation and depression) and some people complain of the drug leaving a bad taste in their mouth after use. The truth is, almost all drugs taste nasty, so don't ever be surprised when a drug tastes bad. Be surprised when one actually tastes good!

Long-acting Beta Agonists are inhaled medications that can reduce asthma symptoms for up to 12 hours. They are not used as much as they were in the past, mainly because this type of drug has been determined to cause more severe asthma attacks. This medication should only be used with an inhaled corticosteroid, and should only be used under the direction of your doctor. (http://www.fda.gov/newsevents/newsroom/pressannouncements/ucm200931.htm)

Combination inhalers have long-acting beta agonists and a corticosteroid in the same inhaler. Use the same cautions with this type of drug as with the long-acting beta agonists. (Symbicort and Dulera are examples of the combination inhalers.)

There are also treatments for people who have allergy-induced asthma. These folks sometimes get help with drugs that suppress the effects of the allergies on their immune system. These therapies are designed to help in several ways and may include allergy shots, allergy medications (antihistamines and decongestants with steroids and/or nasal sprays), or drugs that decrease the immune system's reaction to allergens (Xolair, delivered by injection). (http://www.mayoclinic.com/health/exercise-induced-asthma/DS01040/DSECTION=treatments-and-drugs)

The one big takeaway you should get from this chapter is you can still be in control of your health, even if you have a breathing problem! In fact, if you suffer from a breathing problem, you should be the one person who is in control. Don't let anyone (except a doctor) tell you what to do for your health. If you stay informed and make the right decisions, you'll have a much better life!

...if you suffer from a breathing problem, you should be the one person who is in control. Don't let anyone (except a doctor) tell you what to do for your health.

Action Plan for Breathing Easy

1. Make sure you understand what ***causes*** your symptoms. Once you understand the cause, you will make much better choices about treatment and prevention measures!
2. Consult with your doctor and have a clear result in mind. Think, "I want to be able to play golf without gasping for breath." Having a result in mind before your visit will give you both a common goal. If he/she doesn't think your goal is attainable, find out why and get a second or third opinion. If everyone is in agreement, you'll need to adjust your goal.
3. Make sure you understand what your medicines do! Don't take anyone's advice except your doctor's, and make sure he/she knows everything you take and when you take it! Then, ***do your own research and confirm how the medicine works on you!*** Remember, we are all different; some people react to medicines or combinations of medicines in different ways. Just because a side effect is listed as uncommon doesn't mean you won't get it!
4. Make sure you take all of your health factors into account! Older people and young people need different doses of medicine and, after awhile you may develop a resistance or tolerance to a drug that used to work!
5. If your condition gets worse, ***know when to get help!*** Remember the ABCs of health! Airway, Breathing and Circulation. Your airway and your breathing are vital, and are the first systems to be treated in an emergency for a reason!

6

Back Pain and Muscular Problems

Back pain and muscular problems are very common complaints people suffer from as they age. Depending on the source, there are anywhere from 640 to 850 distinct muscles in the body. (*The American Medical Association Encyclopedia of Medicine*, pp. 703-6; Brandreth, Gyles. *Your Vital Statistics*, p. 17; Cody, John. *Visualizing Muscles*, p. 5.) There is some disagreement as to how to count the muscles, but this is not important in our quest for health.

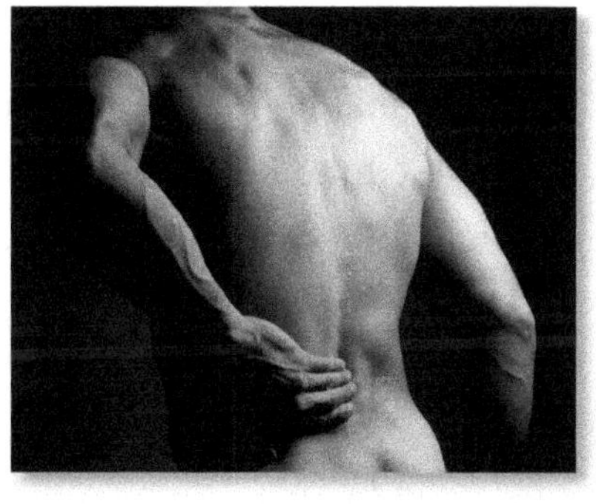

The most important organ in your body is your brain. It controls and coordinates every function of your body, even down to the function of the individual cells. Your brain is surrounded by a hard, bony covering (the skull) that completely protects the delicate tissue of the brain.

The skull is made up of several plates of bone that are connected together and form a hole at the bottom which is called the foramen magnum. This is where the spine begins. The brain feeds into the brainstem (which controls the most important organs of your body), and then into the spinal cord further down your neck.

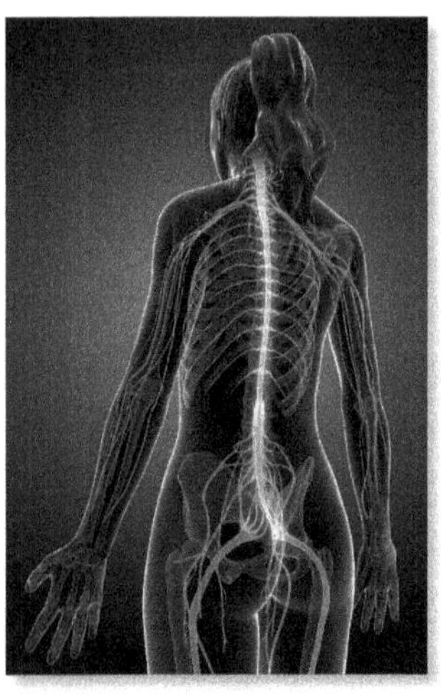

The back is composed of three connected areas. The neck or cervical spine has seven bones which connect at your shoulders to the mid-back or thoracic spine. The thoracic spine has 12 bones and the ribs attach to these bones to protect the vital organs (heart, lungs, liver, etc.) of your body. The lower back or lumbar spine is comprised of five bones and is connected to the base of the spine (the sacrum), which sits between the pelvis or the hips.

The spinal bones (for the most part) have a central round part in front called the body, which is connected to pieces of bone on the side of the body (called lamina) which are fused into the "bump" you feel in the middle of your back, called the spinous process. The spinous process and the lamina form a central canal that protects the spinal cord.

Most of your body weight is supported in the spine through the joints of the spine which link the bone above with the one below. These joints are called the uncinate processes, and they give you the strength and support to allow smooth movement. (http://www.eorthopod.com/content/low-back-pain)

Between each of the bones in the spine is a cushion called a disc which literally absorbs the force as you move. The disc has two parts, a softer center part (called the nucleus), and a tough outer ring (the annulus fibrosis). The discs keep the bones of the spine apart and help form an opening for the spinal nerves to exit on the side of the spine. This is an important point, because if the discs get damaged or bulge, this may irritate the spinal nerves and result in pain! (http://www.mayoclinic.com/health/bulging-disk/AN00272)

One of the main reasons people experience back pain is because the spinal nerves get irritated. Your spine protects the spinal cord and the delicate nerves of the body, which transmit information from your brain to every organ and system in your body.

The spinal cord is attached to the brain at the base of your skull and sends branches of nerves out through the spinal openings to allow the spinal nerves to touch every part of your body in order to regulate each and every cell on a minute-to-minute basis.

Your brain records everything you do from moving to thinking, and this record is stored in your brain. This is how you are able to do complex motions like walking and driving without giving it much thought! The brain has pathways that learn and are activated by daily activities to create "muscle memory." (http://lifehacker.com/5799234/how-muscle-memory-works-and-how-it-affects-your-success)

This is why some people have horrible posture (which is very hard to correct) and others have beautiful, upright posture that allows them to easily carry themselves through life. Posture is not inherited, it is learned! But, if your mother or father has a bad way of carrying themselves, you learn this posture from an early age and correcting it can be very difficult. This learned behavior is so embedded in your brain that it may be difficult to change unless you make a dedicated effort to change it!

If the spine is in proper position, the openings formed by the bones and the discs are large enough to allow the nerves to pass out to the body and every impulse from your brain passes efficiently and cleanly to the organs and muscles. When this takes place, your body uses the least amount of energy necessary to function, and you begin to feel like you did when you were younger!

Keeping the nerve system free from irritation is one of the best things you can do to prevent back pain. You will also feel the benefits in other ways. The nerves in your body are damaged by pressure or stretching. This is why you need to be aware of your spine and nerve system, even though you may not be aware of its function.

Your organ systems cannot function without the control your brain and nerve system provide every minute of each day. The result of any damage to this system could be catastrophic and will cause a loss of health, even with minor interference.

You may remember Christopher Reeve. He was the Hollywood actor who played the role of "Superman" in the 1990s. Reeve had a fall from a horse in 1995, which resulted in a broken neck, and the rest of his life he was a quadriplegic from this injury. The point of the story is he only broke two bones in the fall from the horse. Unfortunately, the bones he broke were very high in his neck, which caused him to lose function in his body and, ultimately, cost him his life. (http://www.chrisreevehomepage.com/biography.html)

The nerves in your body come directly from the spinal cord. When you injure the spine at a certain level, the effects of the damage can be severe and painful. As bad as this sounds, the real problem is the loss of organ function. When the spine is injured, the resulting spinal cord damage may result in a loss of organ function, which would cause disease and could potentially shorten your life!

Common causes of back pain

Damaged or ruptured disc - The disc is the cushion between the bones of the spine and, as mentioned earlier, it forms the opening for the spinal nerve to exit on the side of the spine. When the disc gets injured, it can bulge or herniate, which causes a part of the disc to press on the nerve. For most people, this causes severe pain and prevents them from being able to do everyday activities (called activities of daily living or ADLs).

When the disc gets injured, it can bulge or herniate, which causes a part of the disc to press on the nerve.

The disc injury is not the problem; the nerve pressure is! If the disc bulges out to the front of the spine, then the disc bulging may not cause pain or problems until the person is much older. Then, the normal amount of space between the bones decreases and the degeneration (arthritis) gets worse.

Over time, the loss of space between the bones from this process causes nerve irritation or compression, leading to pain or numbness as the nerve dies from the compressive forces. The symptoms in this type of injury appear slowly over time and, unfortunately, the damage done to the spine and nerves may be irreversible. (http://www.spine-health.com/conditions/herniated-disc/diagnosing-disc-problems)

Spinal stenosis - Spinal stenosis is a condition in the spine which causes pain as a result of narrowing or closing down of the openings where the spinal cord or nerve roots pass through the spinal canal. Some people are born with small openings, and others suffer from narrowing of this space as they age or damage their back. Arthritis may also cause stenosis if it affects the joints in the back area of the spine. (http://www.niams.nih.gov/Health_Info/Spinal_Stenosis/)

The spinal cord divides into spinal nerve roots which pass through the spine and transmit signals from the brain to the rest of the body.

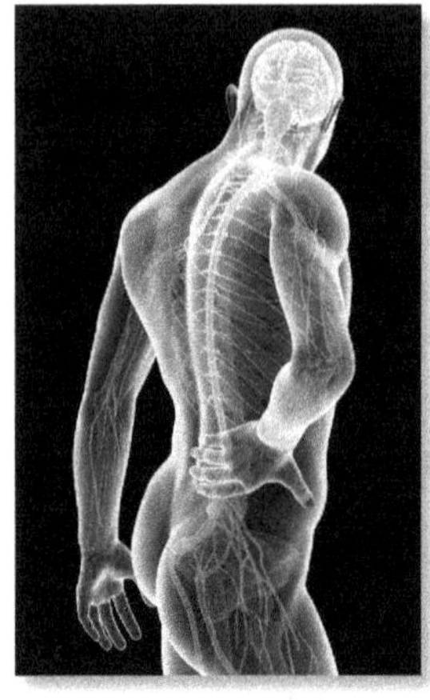

This opening is made up of the borders of the spinal joints (the spinal bone above and below) and the disc. If the space formed by the spinal bones and the disc is too small, the spinal nerve is subject to pressure or stretching when you move or exert. This is the source or cause of your pain.

Unfortunately, there is no pill or procedure which will permanently fix the problem. Spinal stenosis is a difficult problem to manage, but you can decrease your suffering and prevent disability with proper care and rehabilitation. Make sure you do your research and get a program you will continue. Stenosis requires you to take charge for the rest of your life!

Muscle strains - Muscles that attach to the spine help you move in all directions. These muscles may be very large or long (the spinal erectors, or the latissimus muscles), or they may be very small and help you move in only one direction (the multifidus and rotatory muscles). Whatever the size or function of the muscles, they can all be damaged from use or overuse. As we age, we all suffer from muscle loss.

When I was young, there was a man named Jack LaLanne who was one of the best fitness experts in the U.S. Mr. LaLanne was on TV ***all of the time!*** Even when he was older, he found out new ways to pitch products and programs, regarding fitness and health. But as he aged, he didn't look as good as he did when he was young. In fact, I felt he was a bit of a joke…until I started aging! Then I found out just how hard it is to stay in shape as you age!

Even if you work out every day, you will find the aging process is more difficult to overcome! You may even give up your quest for better health through exercise…*don't!* Fitness should be a lifetime goal and pursuit! You must do something to keep your fitness… even if you can only do a little. Fitness is one of those things that is a must, if you intend to live a long life!

I do not want to live the last years of my life in bed or in a wheelchair! I hope you don't, either. That said, what you can do should be the rule of what you will do! Don't look at yourself in the mirror and hate what you see! We are all where we are because of what we have done, and there is ***nothing you or I can do about the past! Don't dwell on it, deal with it!***

Even if you work out every day, you will find the aging process is more difficult to overcome!

Now, let's give you the rules about muscle strains! When muscles contract, the fibers of the muscles pull against each other and they shorten the muscle length, and cause the muscle fibers to bunch up (which gives you that neat little bulge in your biceps). If you damage the muscle, the fibers don't let go after the contraction is completed. This causes a knot to develop which can be painful and cause damage as you age or continue to exercise in spite of the muscle strain.

If the fibers of the muscle don't let go, then the next contraction of the fibers may cause other fibers to get damaged. Before you know it, you have a muscle that appears to be healthy but suddenly tears unexpectedly. This is why you will see highly-trained and conditioned athletes at the Olympics who have run three or four races with no problems who suddenly pull up lame in a later race after pulling a muscle.

So, what do you do about this? These "injured fibers" are actually parts of the muscles that are in a constant state of excitement. They never let go because they can't let go (from the damaged fibers). So, the nerve energy needed to stimulate the muscle is smaller because the nerve system is in a state of constant excitement, which keeps the muscle slightly contracted all the time.

In order to get the muscles to let go so you can feel like you did before the injury, you will need to get the proper type of care! You must also exercise in the right way and prevent injuries in the future. When you do get the occasional injury, if you get the right type of care quickly you will not suffer as long, and you will also be able to return to your lifestyle quickly! This is the one part that most people miss!

There are several different ways to do this. You will need to decide what fits your needs and demands the best! Remember, you can combine these approaches to make a custom solution for your life. Never let anyone convince you that there is only one option for your health!

Options for care for muscular back pain

1. Medically speaking, the first thing offered to almost every patient who has a muscular back problem is fairly standard. Muscle relaxers to reduce muscle spasms and pain-killers to decrease discomfort. So you will likely be asked to try NSAIDs (non-steroidal anti-inflammatory drugs) and/or muscles relaxers (Flexeril-cyclobenzaprine is common). Remember, you may experience the side effects from any drug you take!

   How this works - Muscle relaxers work in a very simple way: the drug dampens the effect of the central nervous system. The net effect of this is the muscle does not respond to the stimulation of the nerve (through the many pathways a nerve may be activated), and this decreases the muscle spasm and the pain which may be caused by the spasm. (http://www.webmd.com/back-pain/muscle-relaxants-for-low-back-pain)

   NSAIDs work by decreasing the swelling of the soft tissues of the body (muscles are soft tissue) which decreases the pressure and pain. NSAIDs also block certain chemicals in the body that alert the body of damage to tissues and cause pain when you get injured. (http://www.medicinenet.com/nonsteroidal_antiinflammatory_drugs/article.htm)

2. Physical therapy (PT) is medical option number two. A therapist will meet with you (usually in their office) and design a program of exercise, stretching, and may use mechanical or electrical machines to help the injured tissues and muscles heal faster. PTs may also use stretching or massage to stabilize the injured areas and restore more normal function to the tissues.

   How it works - There are a lot of opinions on how PT actually works, and there are a lot of people and professionals who have good and bad things to say regarding PT. The truth is, you need to determine if PT is for you! The physical therapist will follow the doctor's orders and will treat only what the doctor tells him/her to treat.

   Rehabilitation of injuries and after surgery is really where PT shines. Most excellent PTs use a variety of exercises to strengthen injured areas and promote long-term healing in your body. If the rehabilitation therapy doesn't work, you need to report this to the doctor and the PT. (http://www.spine-health.com/wellness/exercise/rehabilitation-and-exercise-following-spine-surgery).

3. Chiropractic care works wonderfully for back pain and muscle strains of almost all types. The truth is, the chiropractic profession is the second largest health care provider, and it is one of the most effective forms of care with little or no side effects.

   Chiropractors treat muscle strains and back pain with gentle, effective adjustments that remove nerve irritation and speed the healing process. Millions of people get adjusted and find the relief to be lasting. Today, more professional athletes get chiropractic care than ever before to get that "little edge" they need to perform at their best!

How it works - Chiropractic care works by removing interference to the nerve system. Your doctor will evaluate your problem with a physical examination and may take x-rays to determine exactly where you have a spinal problem. If needed, he/she will give you specific adjustments to your spine and may work with the damaged muscles to make sure you have the best chance of healing. Some chiropractic doctors refer to PTs or MDs and many will use therapy much like the PT to help you feel better fast!

4. Active Release Technique is a soft-tissue management system delivered by certified providers who have been trained and have passed the certification test for each area of the body. These trained and certified providers are more than capable to handle almost any muscular problem in almost any patient. You may have guessed from this paragraph that I am an ART certified provider! I have not only witnessed the "miracles" of chiropractic, but I have also been told many times that I am a "wizard who knows just where to work." This is due in part to the training and the excellent preparation I received from my ART training. If ART doesn't work, you may be sure that your problem ***requires medical attention!*** It is, without a doubt, one of the best treatments available for any type of muscular problem! (http://www.activerelease.com/)

   How it works - ART works by precision. The provider will ask you how you injured yourself and ask for your input to make the treatment work more effectively. If fully certified, he/she may ask you to do specific movements to help the treatment, and will use pressure in the area of injury to get rid of the adhesion that is causing your problem. You will very likely feel a "burn" as the treatment is performed, but you should be in control of how much pain you feel.

After care, most patients report they "feel lighter." Active Release Technique should be provided by ***certified practitioners only***. These providers have been trained and have passed tests to become certified in different areas of the body, and maintain their certification on a yearly basis. This is important because the technique is constantly being updated. If you get ART from a person who claims to know it but is not certified, you should look for another provider who ***is certified!*** This will give you the best chance of getting the best care for your money!

5. Massage therapy works for some people as a stand-alone option. This type of therapy is well known by most people. Massage works by releasing the tension people feel when muscles become stressed or strained. The therapist uses their hands, and sometimes other tools or other techniques, to remove or reduce the tension in the injured tissues.

   How it works - Sessions usually last from ten minutes to hours, with the most common time frame of about one hour for most sessions. You need to be clear about what type of massage you want, and be careful to direct the therapist for the best results! There have been many sessions where I left a bit upset because the therapist did not do what I wanted, or did not understand what I wanted during the session. Communication is the key to better results!

6. Spinal injections may help to reduce the inflammation and pain, or your doctor may offer you bracing or surgery to correct the problem. Please be educated when these services are offered. Your doctor/caregiver should ask you to show them where you hurt, to clarify any other medical problems or procedures you

have had, and if you are on any medications or are allergic to any drugs.

How it works - Injections work by placing drugs (usually anesthetics and steroids) through a needle into the area around an injured nerve root (epidural steroid injection), or into a trigger point (a spasming muscle group). These shots are usually effective in getting rid of pain, but you may need other types of care as follow-up.

Some doctors will use a brace to help a patient who has back pain. Braccs havc many different forms and some even have elastic parts that surround metal stays, which help take the pressure off of the back or the injured joint. While wearing a brace, you need to make sure you don't do too much work, because the brace may actually make you feel stronger. This is not the case, and we have seen many patients who injured themselves worse while wearing a brace.

Although bracing may shorten the time and duration of your pain, wearing a brace improperly may prolong the time you need to recover. Make sure you get a brace that will work for you in the way you want it to work. We have seen many people who come in with a brace that does not fit or does not help them when they work. They basically wasted their money and their time.

We also offer our patients relief with a TENS unit. This electrical machine sends a signal into the muscles and tissues of the back, creating a block to some or all of the pain fibers. It decreases the pain in most patients and helps to reduce the amount of drugs a patient with back pain will need to use to be comfortable.

Obviously, I have not offered ***every type*** of care for back pain or muscle strain, but the most common types of care are here! Also, these types of care are the most effective and the most commonly used. That said, you need to decide what type of care is best for you! Don't let anyone dictate the type of care you get...***for any reason you consider important!***

If you are suffering from the effects of a spinal injury, your options get more complex. You will often be told that you will need or must have surgery to fix a disc that is bulging. This may not be true if the disc bulge is small. However, we have seen many patients who have a small bulge, but also have small openings where the nerves exit the spine. In this case, you may need disc surgery for a small disc bulge.

When I first began practice, we only had x-rays and CT scans to diagnose patients. Then a new imaging technique emerged. The Magnetic Resonance Imaging machine (MRI) was developed, and medical doctors went wild for a very short time. I remember quite clearly many patients who were angry as they told me that their MD apologized to them for not believing they actually had a disc problem (remember the "It's all in your head" line?).

Then an MRI confirmed what the doctor had never thought was possible! Many of these "head cases" actually had a problem that could not be seen by standard medical tests of the day. The doctors literally got caught by this new imaging science and hundreds, if not thousands, of people who suffered from back pain were now told they actually had a problem that was missed.

Now the MRI is so commonplace that the doctors who read the MRI studies (radiologists) don't think a disc bulge of three millimeters is a big deal! So now the tests are evolving further. We now have standing MRIs across the country. Now we can see how a patient's body reacts to the force of gravity, and we can see if their disc can overcome that force in a standing position!

But we still have many other problems that we must consider. How do the tests and the techniques used in surgery actually affect a patient over the rest of their life? This is a question you should really be aware of when you are searching for a cure or relief from your pain.

You must look at several issues...how do you spend your days? If you had to, could you or would you change your profession to avoid re-injury? Do you understand all of the factors and stresses you subject your body and the injured part of your body to on a daily/weekly/monthly basis? Are you willing to accept the changes that will more than likely be permanent after your surgery?

We had a patient who had one surgery for lower back pain and had to use a walker for the rest of her life! This is not a common event, but it does happen! Over the years of practice, I have sent several patients to the surgeon because I could not help them meet their goals after an injury. Only one was better after surgery! The rest of those patients felt the same or were worse as a result of the surgery!

My point here is simple. Make sure you consider ***all options and the possible outcomes before any type of therapy!*** As a Nurse Practitioner, I always tell my patients the side effects of any drug I order before I give them the drug! As a chiropractor, I would constantly tell my patients that chiropractic was a great service, but it did not always work for every patient and there were risks in getting adjusted (even though the risks are small)!

The big difference is, once you get surgery you can never get

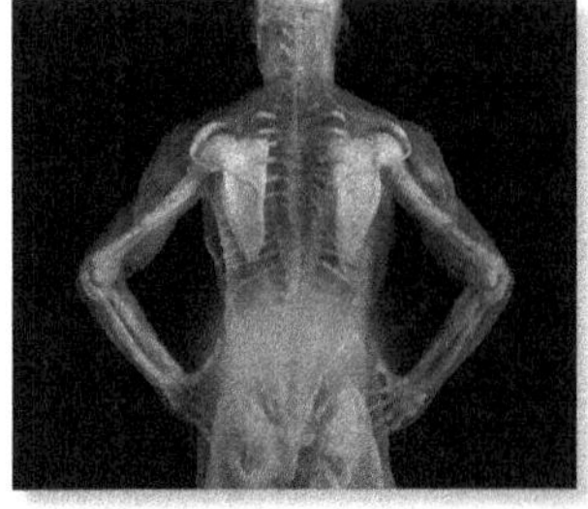

uncut! Most of my faithful patients understand that they must take the lead role in their health care if they want to be in control of the results of their care and the outcome of their life! This is a big concept that a lot of people in medicine (especially the patients) don't get! Patients often think they can just show up with a problem and the doctor/ surgeon will fix it, when or if it gets bad enough. Nothing could be further from the truth!

...once you get surgery you can never get uncut!

Action Plan for Back Problems

1. If you have a back problem, the number one thing you must do is **rest**. I have personally injured myself worse after hurting my back because I could not rest.
2. There are many risks when you try to treat your own back pain. If you have a disc injury, you could make things much worse and suffer more. Ice is always a good place to start, but if ice makes your pain worse, stop using it quickly. Bracing your back to add support is a great idea. I wear a brace in my office to prevent injuries.
    a. Get to the doctor ASAP and get a diagnosis for your pain. If you can, use NSAIDs or aspirin to help decrease your pain. Hot or cold patches may dull your pain, but do not take someone else's medication for pain. I have treated patients who thought a loved one's medication would work, but suffered serious side effects from the drug!
3. I recommend trying chiropractic first, physical therapy or medicine second, and surgery is always the last option for back problems. Remember, you can never get uncut from surgery.
4. If chiropractic, physical therapy and medication don't work (or only work for a short time), you need to get an MRI of the injured part of your back to make sure you do not have an injured disc. If you do, you need the help of an expert surgeon.
5. If you have back surgery, you will need to rehabilitate your back. Make sure your weight stays in an ideal range and continue to help yourself with regular exercise to prevent a new injury from occurring.

Muscle Aches and Pains

Muscle aches and pains come from several different causes. Your muscles are actually made up of fibers. The fibers are made of myofibrils, which are made up of the proteins called actin and myosin. These proteins are the building blocks of the muscle and when they contract, they literally "bunch up," which causes the bulge in a muscle.

The muscle fibers are insulated from each other, and are activated by the electrical impulses from the nerve system which is controlled by your brain. So, we are back to the basis of control, which is in your brain! (Ever wonder why the doctor tells you, "It's all in your head"?) So, when you decide you want to learn a new dance step, or you want to play golf or tennis, your brain works first, and your muscles follow the lead of the impulses sent by your brain!

...when you decide you want to learn a new dance step, or you want to play golf or tennis, your brain works first, and your muscles follow the lead of the impulses sent by your brain!

If you repeat an activity, or if you never release the tension in your muscles from an activity, then your muscles may cramp from the effort. This is caused when the muscle burns energy (called ATP) and produces lactic acid as a result. If enough lactic acid builds up in your muscles, then you will feel the burning sensation that comes from exertion.

The problem with "the burn" is what it does if it builds up over time! We sit all day at desks, and many of us now use a mouse while we work. This doesn't't sound at all stressful, but if you use a mouse most of the day and never move your hand through a full range of motion, you may cause only a specific set of muscles to work hard, and the buildup of lactic acid in a small group of muscles will create symptoms of carpal tunnel from the repeated stress (called a repetitive stress injury). (http://www.emedicinehealth.com/repetitive_motion_injuries/article_em.htm)

There are many activities that can cause this same problem! This is due to the fact that we now have wonderful new technologies that allow us to get things done with minimum effort. However, research has shown us that this minimum effort, if sustained over hours, causes major problems.

If we rarely rest the muscles we use to move a mouse, type, or do other repetitive activities, we get a build-up of lactic acid in the fine muscles and, over time, this causes scarring of the tissues

If we rarely rest the muscles we use to move a mouse, type, or do other repetitive activities, we get a build-up of lactic acid in the fine muscles and, over time, this causes scarring of the tissues. This scarring will cause problems with muscle tissues, and may affect nerve function and cause pain, if not addressed.

If you place a load on the muscles, the fibers get stressed and they react to the stress by growing and adapting to the load to make it easier for you to handle the weight. This process is the muscle's way of making you into a stronger and newer you every time you pick up something heavy! But this is not what a lot of people do today! (http://ed.ted.com/lessons/what-makes-muscles-grow-jeffrey-siegel)

Now that you understand a bit of how muscles work, you need to understand one of the biggest problems we all face when we go to the medical doctor complaining of muscle pain. Medical doctors basically have only a few ways of treating muscle aches or pains! If you have simple pain from exercise, your doctor will probably tell you to ease the pain with rest, ice, and use non-steroidal anti-inflammatory drugs (NSAIDs) like Tylenol or Motrin.

Your doctor may send you for physical therapy if the drugs don't work for your pain. This is not because he/she doesn't care, it is simply because medical doctors are not well-versed on what needs to be done about muscle and joint pain! These types of symptoms, although very common, are not life-threatening, so your doctor will do the simplest thing he can and hope for the best! (http://www.nlm.nih.gov/medlineplus/ency/article/003178.htm)

Options for care

If you injure yourself and you think the injury is due to muscle or joint strain or a sprain, the first thing you should do is rest, ice, compression and elevation (RICE is the acronym). After a few days, if there is ***no severe injury***, we ask patients to use castor oil drizzled on a washcloth, put over the hurt area with a heating pad on ***low heat*** to drive the oil into the skin. (Castor oil decreases swelling naturally.) This works very well for most injuries and even helps bruises heal a bit faster.

1. As said before, your medical doctor has only a few tricks in the bag when it comes to treating muscle strains and pain. You most likely will be offered NSAIDs and painkillers first. When these fail, you will be given a prescription for physical therapy, if it is covered by your insurance company. Please remember that any drug will dull your ability to feel pain and you could injure yourself or make the problem worse while under the influence of the drug!

   Unfortunately, physical therapy doesn't work well for these types of injuries in all cases. Some people will get better with physical therapy, some will stay the same, and others will get worse. You must control your outcome by getting involved with the type of care you get, reporting how the care works, and making sure your care is adjusted to your needs to get the best outcome!

We have seen many cases where the physical therapist has done what they felt was right for the patient, but the patient did not respond well to the care, and the result was the patient gave up or did not return to complete the necessary care. This is one of the biggest problems in providing care for patients! As a provider, we sometimes don't know how the patient feels and most of us cannot read minds. This is why you must report your personal experience to your caregiver on a daily basis.

If the physical therapy does not work, the doctor may try steroid injections and then he is left with surgery. Surgery is not really a good choice for muscle pain unless you have torn a muscle and it needs to be reattached. If this happens to a muscle or a tendon, be assured that the surgery is necessary in most cases and the medical doctor is the ***only choice for this type of care!***

How this works - NSAIDs and other drugs work by decreasing swelling in the injured muscles and tissues and providing pain relief to the patient. Physical therapy works by using exercise, stretching and massage to get the soreness out of the area and strengthen the injured area to restore function and prevent injury in the future.

2. Active Release Technique (ART) is not recommended universally by all health care providers, but it should be! As a Certified ART provider, I can tell you that I am prejudiced regarding this type of care, but you can do your own research and decide for yourself if this is the best type of care for your problem! (www.activerelease.com)

   ART works by getting to the core of the injury and removing

the main cause of the problem. The provider will ask you how you got injured, ask you to move the injured area while he/she feels for the source of the pain or problem, and then he will work the injured area in the best way possible to make the muscle fibers move independently, which helps your body heal!

After your treatment is complete, you should perform specific stretches daily to help the injured area remain free from any scarring/adhesions. This also helps make your body stronger and less likely to be injured in the future! If your care is not progressing, your ART provider will suggest a different method, or he may let you know that you need further evaluation or tests to determine if you need a different type of care.

We had a specific case in our office that illustrates this point. I tell almost every patient (I try to tell them all) that if ART doesn't work, then they have a deeper problem that will need another type of care. A young man had hurt his hip in an accident where he was running away from another person in a flag football game. They tried to catch him, but, they were only able to grab him by the top of his foot. He pulled away, but was injured in the incident.

We worked for weeks on his hip but he never got completely better, and was unable to run at top speed without re-injury or pain. As a result, we told his mother that we felt he needed an MRI. After this was done, the tumor that was causing his problem was found! His mother told us that we were the only office that suggested he get an MRI.

This also illustrates why you must stay involved in your care and how your outcome can be directed when getting proper care! The young man's life was changed by this recommendation! He would have had to live with the pain and would not have been able to return to his active life without the surgery that removed the tumor which caused the pain in his hip!

How ART works - ART works by finding the specific nerves, muscles and fibers that are injured. The provider then uses his/her hands and possibly other types of tools to brace or hold against the injured area and force the injured tissue to pull through the contact point established by the provider. It literally helps your body heal by unknotting the knotted area and allows new, "normal" tissue to replace injured fibers. (www.activerelease.com)

3. Acupuncture sometimes works very well for muscular problems. There are different types of acupuncturists, so please know what you want and like before you select the doctor who performs your acupuncture! I went to a very highly-recommended doctor in Austin, Texas, after I pulled my hamstring waterskiing. The pain was so bad it kept me from sleeping for many nights, and I had problems walking during the day without a noticeable limp. This doctor came in and put needles into my leg exactly where it hurt!

Unfortunately, the pain got worse with the needles. I complained and he told me, "Oh, don't be such a baby, the pain will go away soon!" I can tell you that the only thing that went away was me! I also made it a point to tell anyone who asked about my experience what the doctor said. I don't normally try to steer patients away from particular doctors, but in this case, I felt totally justified!

This is not a typical encounter! There are many excellent doctors who do a great job with acupuncture, and I have practiced the art for more than 30 years. I am simply pointing out how you need to be in control, even when you seek care that is not ***universally practiced in the US!*** Do not tolerate bad care or service in any form! If you do, expect to be disappointed regularly by your health care providers!

How acupuncture works - Acupuncture is based on very ancient Asian medicine systems which were charted by "physicians" in the Chinese dynasties. These doctors usually had to pass this information down to their sons and daughters (usually the son) who would improve on the information used to heal or create a desired effect for the patient.

The needles or pressure points are usually around nerves in the body and the electrical effect of the body does the work. Acupuncture is effective when used properly and done by a ***qualified doctor!***

There are many people who claim to have a knowledge of this type of medicine without being properly trained. This is because there are states where the education requirements are very relaxed. If done properly, the treatment should be comfortable (after a short time) and the effects can be quite long-lasting.

There are many different ways to get a result using acupuncture. The needles alert the body of an area that needs stimulation or a calming of energy. The body will interpret the need and use the needles as a conduit to create the needed toning or calming of energy, which may help the patient heal.

4. Exercise is used by many people. However, if you are already injured, exercise will ***usually not make your injury better.*** People are under the impression that exercise is what physical therapists do, so they think they can exercise without the direction of a qualified PT and get the same results. I have had many patients over the years tell me, "I hurt myself working out, so I just thought I needed to change the workout and it would go away!"

Nothing is worse than doing something you think will help, and finding out that you have made your condition worse as a result! Exercise is actually not the thing to do after an injury! If you continue to work out in spite of an injury, you may make things much worse.

I had a very athletic man come into the office who was trying to get into the best shape of his life. He told me how much weight he was lifting during his exercise sessions and I asked him, "Are you planning on competing in a body-building competition?" He told me, "No, I just want to get better in all areas of my life!"

Well, he was lifting what I considered was an ***insane amount of weight*** during his workouts. I asked him to back off a bit and he refused, even though I told him that I thought he might get injured from the effort (he was already getting care for his back pain from exercise).

The result was he herniated a disc in his lower back trying to do a maximum effort lift while squatting! He had surgery, and he could never reach the goals he set for himself in the future. I believe that exercise is essential, but only to moderate discomfort! Extreme discomfort during exercise is almost always the signal of an injury!

How it works - Exercise works by making the body stronger. You may need help when you begin exercising! If you don't have a solid idea of how you should use exercise to help your specific problem, get help from a ***certified trainer!*** You will most certainly get the benefit of this expertise. Certified trainers can help you get started and may be able to help you prevent an injury, which can save you more pain and the possibility of surgery.

Action Plan for Muscle Injuries

1. Make sure you know why your back or muscles hurt. If you injured yourself during exercise or activity, remember RICE (Rest, Ice, Compression, and Elevation) for the first three days after an injury. Use the best braces or supports to prevent further injury to your back or joints.
2. Know your options for care when you get injured. Get advice from a qualified medical or chiropractic professional and follow the advice!
3. Take advantage of the newer technologies to make sure you get the correct diagnosis (MRI and CT scans). Do everything you can to avoid an unnecessary surgery (of any type).
4. Try Active Release Technique, massage and exercise to rehabilitate the injury (if possible). A lot of injuries that required surgery in the past do not get surgery today! Explore your options and make sure to follow through with the care and the advice of your chosen experts. Use the Internet for research and make sure to select care that will meet your goals.
5. Don't begin with exercise unless you are sure or are told exercise will help your injury! Get more than one opinion for any injury that requires surgery, and make sure you research every kind of care before paying for help! This will save you thousands of dollars, and prevent needless suffering caused by the wrong treatment.

7
Weight Problems

I have written about weight problems and the dangers of carrying too much weight before. I am writing a bit more here. Some of this information may repeat, but it is too important to miss, and some people will jump to this section without reading the book in order.

You must do all you can to make sure you get the best out of your life! There is new information from studies on weight. This information speaks to the heart of why we can't lose weight.

What was discovered, in part, was that sitting in a chair all day may be one of the most common things we do that will shorten your life! You must move your body (exercise) in order to lose weight, and you must have a general level of fitness in order to move your body. (http://news.health.com/2012/10/08/whats-the-best-workout-for-weight-loss/)

Find a type of exercise you will do regularly, and the battle of the bulge is half won! In order to lose weight effectively, you need to find a way to stay motivated. This means you need exercise that you will do or enjoy doing regularly.

Take care of your body, keep your weight in check, and this will prevent the diseases that you may be genetically programmed for, in spite of your genetic tendency for a disease! There is nothing your doctor can do, no matter how great he/she is, to stop you from hurting yourself from poor lifestyle choices, or genetic traits but you can!

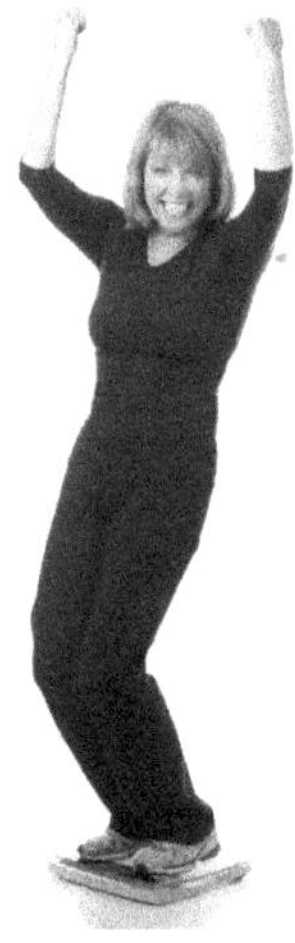

Choose the path you want for yourself and your family, then go for it! Don't let anyone tell you that your weight/lifestyle goal can't be attained! There are literally thousands of people who make their dreams come true in spite of huge odds, and you can, too!

Even your genetics may be overcome if you remain dedicated and work hard! There are programs that explain just how easily this can be done, and it doesn't take a lifetime to make an impact on your health! (www.kpbs.org/news/2013/apr/08/truth-about-exercise-michael-mosley/)

Exercise and stretching need to be a part of every exercise plan. If you need guidance or help to get started, ask your doctor what you are able to do. The other option is to go to a local gym, look on the Internet, or simply buy a beginning program from a local store and get started. Start slowly and be careful! Especially if you are new to exercise, or have not exercised in a while, you must start with gentle exercise! (www.fitnessblender.com)

I have had many patients over the years ask me how to exercise, and every single patient has to start in a different way. The most impressive thing I have seen was a woman who had not exercised for years. I really think she had never exercised in her life, but that may not be the case.

She asked me how she could start (she was a very large, out of shape woman). I simply asked her what she was ***willing to do reg-***

ularly. Her answer shocked me, but she was honest. She told me, "I don't like any type of exercise, but I'm willing to do anything you recommend as long as I won't hurt myself and I don't have to sweat!"

I had never heard anyone express such limitations! Especially since I told her she was getting very close to the point of "no return," where she may never be able to be healthy! I thought about her request for literally weeks and here is what I told her to do…she was to get in a pool and walk for thirty minutes a day during the summer.

She looked at me and laughed! She told me that she didn't know how to swim and didn't think this was a good idea. Then I explained to her the secret of the program…

1. She didn't need any special equipment or training…she could use the local community pool and she already knew how to walk.
2. She wouldn't have to sweat because she would walk in the pool and the water would keep her cool as she exercised.
3. She could do this as long as she wanted and as long as the pool was open.
4. The water would give her body a lift (buoyancy) and this would take the stress off her joints so she could walk farther and increase her exercise without stress or pain.\
5. She was to stay in the shallow end of the pool and only walk… this would ease her fear of the water and she didn't need to know how to swim.
6. The water actually provided a form of resistance that would help her lose weight and build muscle that she desperately needed, and would reduce the daily pain she suffered from aging and lack of exercise!

The results of this "experiment" were amazing! She loved the exercise and lost 40 pounds over the summer. This lady now enjoys a more active and healthy life from doing one simple thing differently! This is an example we can all follow! Your exercise should be a part of your new lifestyle and it must involve movement!

If you looked at the link provided earlier in this section, you know that the one thing most of us do today is sit! We sit and use our computers, we sit and eat, we sit and watch TV. Our grandparents didn't sit as much as we do. Their parents sat even less!

Sitting most of the day will cause you to lose your muscle tone and will make you unhealthy for life! If you want to be healthy, you must move every day! We now have research that proves that if you sit at work for 6-8 hours, even if you go to the gym for an hour every day, you may still have problems staying fit. New research done by researchers at Queen's University Belfast states that sitting is as bad for your back as smoking is for your lungs! (http://www.irishtimes.com/news/health/study-shows-prolonged-sitting-as-bad-as-smoking-for-health-1.2321802)

This is really bad news because many of us now must sit to work, and this trend is getting worse, not better! Look again at the report and look at the research that supports the idea that the most dangerous thing you may face in your life is a chair! (http://www.kpbs.org/news/2013/apr/08/truth-about-exercise-michael-mosley/)

Other Weight-Related Diseases

There are other diseases that are related to weight, or are caused by weight. If your problem is too much weight, then the two most common problems are Type II diabetes and hypothyroidism.

Type II diabetes is a disease that most people know. It is caused by too much sugar in the blood. This may be the result of genetic programming in your cells, or it may be caused by eating incorrectly and not taking care of your body for years. Type II diabetes is described in detail later in the book.

Thyroid disorders are weight problems related to an over-active or, more commonly, an under-active thyroid. Thyroid disorders are an undiagnosed epidemic according to several authorities. There may be as many as 20-60 million people with thyroid disease, and many of these people are undiagnosed. (http://www.thyroid.org/media-main/about-hypothyroidism/)

Hypothyroidism is a condition where your thyroid doesn't put out enough thyroid hormone. This will affect literally every cell in your body! The thyroid is a small organ of the endocrine system that sits in the middle part of your neck below your Adam's apple. Hypothyroidism may be triggered by an infection that attacks your thyroid (Hashimoto's thyroiditis) or other autoimmune/degenerative problems. (http://www.mayoclinic.org/diseases-conditions/hashimotos-disease/basics/definition/con-20030293)

Your thyroid is controlled by your pituitary gland (at the base of your brain). When your pituitary gland produces thyroid-stimulating hormone (TSH), your thyroid produces T4 (thyroxine), which gets converted into T3 in the blood. This hormone affects your metabolism, your immunity, and your bone density. The thyroid produces a very small amount (about one teaspoon) of thyroid hormone per year.

The thyroid is vital to your health and has been linked to over 50 diseases. Many of these diseases are deadly (cancer, heart disease, obesity…) and impact the lives of those who are affected. Most of the signs and symptoms of thyroid dysfunction are subtle, and cannot be diagnosed without the help of a medical expert! (http://thyroid.about.com/od/symptomsrisks/a/Why-Are-So-Many-People-Getting-Thyroid-Disease.htm)

There are things you can do to make sure you do not develop full-blown thyroid disease. If you have hypothyroidism, you develop a low body temperature, have problems losing and maintaining your weight (even with diet and exercise), and you have chronic low energy. You can screen yourself at home by taking your temperature and keeping a food diary to see if your weight gain is due to dietary issues.

You may also notice a thickening and drying of your skin and nails, swelling of your tongue (macroglossia), and breaking, brittle hair. There may also be changes in your immunity to other diseases.

When this happens, it will affect how you feel and how your body reacts to your environment. There are a lot of other problems associated with hypothyroidism. If you think you fit the profile, seek out an expert in your area and get tested! (http://thyroid.about.com/cs/hypothyroidism/a/checklist.htm)

Make sure that your doctor tests you for ***all*** of the necessary things to properly diagnose a low thyroid. According to experts, you will need TSH, T4 (free and total), T3 (free and total), reverse T3, thyroglobulin/thyroid binding hormone, thyroid peroxidase antibodies, and levels for vitamins B and D. These should be done with the other blood studies to make sure you have a thyroid condition.

The reason you want all of these tests is because there may be a good chance that your thyroid will appear normal to the doctor if you do not get the additional testing. This is the reason some experts claim that hypothyroidism is very badly *under-diagnosed in America.* (http://www.drbrownstein.com/)

Hyperthyroidism is a disease where your thyroid produces too much thyroid hormone which causes a lot of other problems. When you have too much thyroxine in your blood, your metabolism speeds up. This can cause sudden weight loss, difficulty sleeping, rapid heartbeat, increased appetite, sensitivity to heat, sweating, changes in bowel patterns, swelling in your neck (goiter), fine, brittle hair, and changes in your skin. (http://www.mayoclinic.org/diseases-conditions/hyperthyroidism/basics/symptoms/con-20020986)

Most of us who have weight problems think that having a problem where we could eat a lot and never gain weight would be great. However, this disease (Grave's) causes thyroid dysfunction, which comes with other things we don't want. It may result in heart damage (rapid heartbeat, atrial fibrillation or congestive heart failure), skin changes, brittle bones, and eye problems. (http://www.mayoclinic.org/diseases-conditions/hyperthyroidism/basics/complications/con-20020986)

Hyperthyroidism can be successfully treated, but you will need the help of an expert endocrinologist!

Our daughter had problems with her thyroid when she went off to college. We tried to help her with every type of holistic therapy we could find, but in the end her endocrinologist was the only one who could help. He treated her for just over a year, and the medications corrected her problem and she is now healthy as ever!

This proves that everyone needs help from time to time. We knew where to look and what to try, but we were unable to help our daughter without expert advice. Medicine should be used only when necessary, but you should know when to ask for help and you should follow the direction of a qualified expert when necessary!

Action Plan for Thyroid Problems

1. Look at your symptoms and decide if you think you may have a thyroid problem. Look for the following things to confirm the problem. Do you have: low body temperature; weight gain or loss that does not get better, even with a strict diet; low energy, even with the proper amount of sleep; hair that is falling out for no reason; low or no sex drive; puffiness in the face, tummy and hips; changes in your skin or a noticeable bump or lump in the lower part of your throat? If you do, you will need to check! Remember, the only way to confirm a thyroid problem is a blood test and eventually a scan (MRI or thyroid ultrasound).
2. Make sure you are taking in the right kinds of supplements. You will need to supplement your diet with iodine (salt with iodine doesn't work). We recommend a product called Iodoral, which has a very good source of iodine and is tolerated very well by most people. (https://www.optimox.com/pics/Iodine/opt_Iodoral.htm)
3. Try to adjust your diet and make sure you are getting ***quality nutritious food*** over quantity. Avoid gluten, empty carbs (like bread, white potatoes, pasta and rice), and sugar as much as possible to see if your body will correct on its own. If this does not work, it's time to get help from your doctor.
4. Be prepared with all of your information. Tell your doctor what you have done to correct your problem and how long you have been working to correct the problems. Be very specific about as much of the information as you can. Let him know if you have a family history of thyroid problems and if you were sick before your problem started.

5. Get the blood tests that your doctor recommends. Make sure to ask him/her to include: TSH, T3 and T4 (regular and free), reverse T3, Thyroid peroxidase antibodies (TPOAb), and Thyroglobulin antibodies (TGAb). You may also want other tests recommended by other medical experts to get a complete picture of the function of your thyroid. Please do what your doctor recommends! Your thyroid is vital to your health and well-being! (http://www.drbrownstein.com/)

If you don't have a disease that causes your weight-gain problems, you need a plan to get your weight down and keep it off! There are literally thousands of ways and plans to lose weight. Google weight loss, and see how many hits you get.

I have tried many of the programs and plans to see which were easy and effective ways to lose weight for my patients. No one plan works for every person. That may be why there are so many plans to choose from.

I really don't like plans that make you buy products to raise your metabolism (how fast you burn calories) or meal replacement plans. The reason I am not a fan, even though these plans will work, is you can get trapped in a loop where you can't lose weight without buying product.

No matter who you are, if you are forced to buy a product to lose weight, you will eventually gain back the weight you lost. We use a medically-supervised weight-loss program that requires little exercise and uses human hormones to speed the weight loss (HCG). This program was developed by a medical doctor and has decades of success and research behind it.

This program helps almost everyone. The only reason a person would not be able to use the diet is if they have had an allergy to the hormone, or if they have had a tumor that was hormone-driven (male or female). Many of our patients tell us they are not hungry at all on this protocol, and they report the program pays for itself in the savings from food they don't buy while losing weight!

You could use other weight-loss programs. There are literally hundreds of them out there with untold success stories. Use the program that you think will give you the best success, and remember that the real problem with weight is what you eat.

Americans eat a diet that is horrible for the body and causes weight gain (even in children). We drive our bodies to the limit with stress and consume food that burns quickly, but leaves an imprint on our future by driving insulin levels high and setting the table for Type II diabetes in the future.

We educate our patients during the weight-loss program to give them the control they must have to avoid the "rebound gain" that sometimes happens when people try to lose weight. We also give them the tools necessary to keep weight in control for a lifetime!

Meal replacement programs are programs that require a person to buy pre-packaged or pre-made meals instead of learning how to eat, them-selves. The real problem we see in patients who have weight problems is they eat without really being hungry, and this causes them to eat more calories than they need to maintain their desired weight.

Over years of problem eating, weight gain becomes the norm. We also know that as we age, we don't need to eat as many calories per day. Yet most Americans still eat about the same amount of calories as they age. This causes mature adults to be overweight and may cause thyroid problems and Type II diabetes.

Weight problems can only be corrected when the person takes control of their diet and their attitude towards food. Knowing what to do when others won't help or don't help you obey the rules is a part of the solution. Make plans to help you succeed even when events and holidays give you an "easy reason" to cheat.

I was very careful to tell my patients about all of the upcoming holidays and events that might give them a hard time during their weight-loss programs. Then a friend of mine told me a very wise thing. He said, "David, there will always be an excuse to cheat if you look for one!" I agreed completely with this, and now I share his wisdom with every person who begins a weight-loss program.

The most honest thing you can do for yourself is start realizing the people who are near (and some who are dear) to you may not really help you lose weight! They will probably ask you if you are sure you really want to lose weight, and you should plan on ways to refuse food when offered.

The reason people gain weight after they lose weight is very simple. They go back to the bad habits they had before they lost weight. You will never maintain weight-loss for long if you don't change how you eat! Dietary changes must be permanent to affect your weight or body type. We tell all of our patients that they must avoid fast food and empty carbohydrates ***forever*** if they expect to maintain a change.

Weight Loss Surgery

Weight loss surgery like liposuction, stomach stapling, banding or bypassing, are options that are used for people who are dangerously overweight. You must be screened to get this surgery, and my sincere hope is that you can succeed without resorting to this method. If this is your last option, understand that I have personally seen people who have eaten through gastric bypasses (a very extreme surgery).

Although this may seem really unusual, it's not. One of the most common problems for doctors who perform gastric surgery is the failure rate of patients who simply regain weight after surgery to prevent them from eating too much. If you think this is you, you need professional help from a psychologist or psychiatrist before surgery.

This also emphasizes the real problem for some people is the level of commitment they have. If you are more committed to eating than to your health, then no surgery will fix the problem.

8

Arthritis

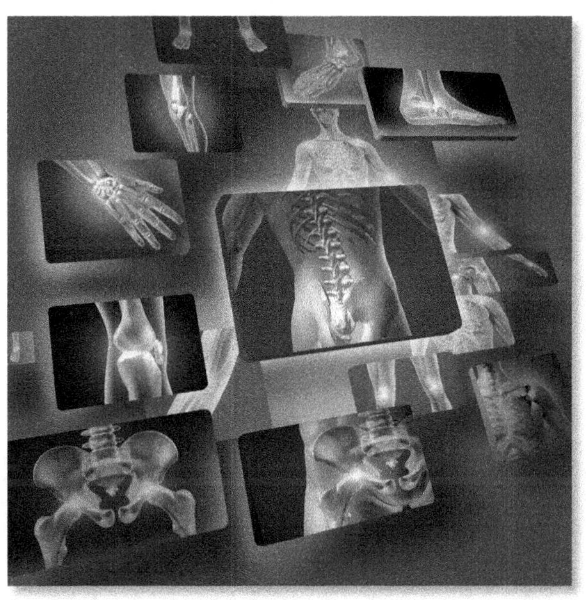

Arthritis is a disease that can rob you of years of life, and even worse, can rob you of the quality of life you want as you age. Arthritis is a condition which can be passed from generation to generation and affects the bones and the joints of the body. Arthritis ***means*** swelling and irritation of a joint or joints. (http://orthopedics.about.com/od/arthritis/f/whatisarthritis.htm)

When you have arthritis, the affected joint can't work properly because the inner surface of the joint, which has cartilage over or between the opposing surfaces, has broken down. This breakdown causes the joint to become misaligned and creates pressure on the inside of the joint that wears the cartilage cushion out faster than normal. The body then responds by forming new bone in the area, and bone spurring is the result.

Bone spurs are basically a defensive mechanism your body uses to prevent injury to an area of weakness. Your body interprets the unstable, rough area as a weak area because it doesn't function normally and it swells from the added stress. This stress causes a response which results in new calcium formation in the area of the stress, and the damaged joint actually fuses (grows together) to prevent motion that is too painful or damaging to the body.

...there are over 100 different types of musculoskeletal conditions which are known to be forms of arthritis.

Arthritis is more than just one disease. In fact, there are over 100 different types of musculoskeletal conditions which are known to be forms of arthritis. Arthritis does not just affect older people.

Juvenile arthritis can be devastating and deadly to young people, and may cause a lifetime of disability and pain to its victims. The most well-known forms of arthritis are osteoarthritis, rheumatoid arthritis, and juvenile arthritis. All different types of arthritis affect the joints of the body in similar ways.

One of the most well-known types of arthritis is **rheumatoid arthritis.** This type of arthritis can cause extreme damage in every area of the body, but it is well known because it affects the hands of the victims and causes a "swan neck deformity" which most of us recognize on sight. Rheumatoid arthritis (RA) may also be diagnosed from a blood test when rheumatoid factor is discovered.

One of the first signs of rheumatoid arthritis is swelling of the joints in most patients. This swelling starts when the immune system malfunctions and begins attacking normal healthy tissue. This attack is the beginning of the disease process, which progresses until the joints are destroyed completely. The worst cases of this type of arthritis lead to severe limitation and disability in patients who have RA.

RA can get so bad that the victim becomes totally disabled and has to use a wheelchair or other device to move. In this stage, the person affected by RA has constant pain and any movement can be difficult and painful. The joints of the body don't function normally and usually fuse as a result of the disease.

Why does this happen?

The most direct and simple answer is... no one knows. RA is one of those diseases that you get from an auto-immune response that is basically out of control. Your body thinks the tissues it is attacking are unhealthy or damaging to your health, and the normal defense system we have inside to protect us kicks in and takes over. Unfortunately, if we ever did find a way to shut this system down, you would get very sick from other causes (given the fact that this system attacks and kills bacteria and other things you are constantly exposed to).

RA is one of those diseases that you get from an auto-immune response that is basically out of control.

The joints in your body have a system that is both fluid and solid to keep the joints functioning and moving smoothly. This system is made up of the bones, which are hard; the cartilage, which is semi-hard and flexible; and fluid to lubricate the joint that is held in place by a capsule which surrounds the entire system.

RA attacks musculoskeletal and the immune system. Other things we do make the problem worse. RA is ***not simply a joint disease!*** It is a complex response of your body which is focused in your joints. Understanding this is how you begin to help yourself! You must pay attention to all of the factors that have been identified and do your best to control everything you can control to get the best outcome.

What we know - RA attacks all of the body tissues, causing swelling, fever, and discomfort, which may happen in bouts of more intense activity called flares. Because most people who are affected are women (70%), hormone fluctuation may play a part in flares. Smoking is also known to increase the severity of the pain and swelling from flares, and we know that genetic tendencies play a part in who gets RA.

If you have RA, this information is not new. Hopefully, you have done your research and have taken care to design a program that includes supplements, dietary changes and exercise, to help manage your symptoms. You must look at all of the ways you can help yourself and do one thing at a time with your doctor's help to maximize your results.

...research has shown that if we are sensitive to certain foods, the body will react with swelling, which could make an arthritic person miserable.

Many of us don't think of food as a cause for swelling in the body, but research has shown that if we are sensitive to certain foods, the body will react with swelling, which could make an arthritic person miserable. The problem is that the body can identify the proteins in food as an intruder that needs to be dealt with, and this can set off a cascade of events and cause inflammation in the body. (http://www.nlm.nih.gov/medlineplus/ency/article/000817.htm)

As you can see, there are a lot of things you could do wrong to make your RA symptoms worse. You must do a lot of things right to make the symptoms better. You must try to find a way to make yourself better without drugs, if possible, or with as few drugs as necessary. Exercise is a very important thing that must be a part of your daily regimen to ease the pain of RA.

The rule on exercise is simple…if it hurts to exercise, rest is the best action. If it hurts to rest, but not to exercise, then exercise is the best action. But, if it hurts to ***rest and exercise***, then you should exercise. The reason for this formula is simple. If you hurt with both rest and exercise, the exercise will at least help your muscles support the injured area, which will give you a better long-term picture.

Because RA destroys the joints and the soft tissues of the body, it is very important that you get exercise to help support the joints and prevent further decay of the soft tissues. Moving the joints also helps by moving the fluid in the joints, which will help nourish the remaining cartilage in the joints. This forces nutrition into the joints, which helps keep the remaining cartilage and muscles as healthy as they can be!

We have found that, for many of our patients, a surprising number get great comfort and relief from a very simple and inexpensive therapy which they can easily do at home. We ask them to simply drizzle castor oil on a cloth or old washcloth, and then place the cloth over the painful, swollen area. They use a heating pad on low heat to help move the castor oil into the skin and most find this remedy relieves most, if not all, of their pain. (http://articles.mercola.com/sites/articles/archive/2012/04/28/castor-oil-to-treat-health-conditions.aspx)

Nutrition

Because your body uses the food you eat to build bone, soft tissues and muscle, you must eat the best food you can afford. Be careful to avoid any foods that cause **any irritation in your body!** We have found over the years that people crave foods that actually make them worse if they have an illness.

Comfort foods (foods that make you feel good or foods that taste good) like cookies and chips don't provide good nutrition for the calories you consume. Sugar (especially table sugar) is well known to be a very poor choice, but is consumed by most people in excess. These daily choices are the foundation of your health and can cause you to suffer greatly as you age! (http://ngm.nationalgeographic.com/2013/08/sugar/cohen-text)

If you want a physical test you can do at home, try this…it may seem like a bit of voodoo, but it actually has a scientific foundation and may convince you that something you love is bad for your body, and bad for you! Get a friend to help you by putting different things in small glass containers with caps on top. Put sugar in one container, flour in another, soy in the third, and milk powder in the last. To keep track of the substances, you can put a mark on the bottom of the container or some other mark to let you know what is in each vial.

The secret to the test is you won't actually touch any of the substances! The glass will allow your body to react, but you won't get the same reaction you will experience from eating the substance. Hold one container in your hand (use your weakest hand) and place the container over your heart. Then, try to **lock** your other arm in front of you with your thumb turned up (some people like to make a fist).

Your friend then tries to gently, but quickly, push down on the outstretched arm to see if you can hold the locked position. This is ***NOT*** a trial of strength! A quick, subtle push by your friend is all that is needed to do this test. In the office, I use only two of my fingers to push down on a patient.

If you cannot hold your arm up in a locked position, this indicates that you may have a sensitivity to whatever you are testing, and the substance is not good for you! This actually works to show people how they may be sensitive to different things that they eat and crave every day! I have had many patients who could not lose weight, and after this simple test they quit eating something (usually wheat) that was keeping them from losing the weight because they were sensitive!

Allow me to take a minute here to tell you the difference between a sensitivity and an allergy. A sensitivity to a food or a substance is a reaction in your body that indicates the food/substance does not sit well in your body. A sensitivity is ***not the same as an allergy!*** It may cause some swelling of the tissues, but you will not react with hives, sneezing or itching. Over time, a sensitivity can develop into a full-blown allergy.

An allergy to something is immediate and can be life-threatening! Think of a mosquito bite and how you get that bump under your skin that itches and stings. This is an allergy! (Most people, about 99%, are allergic to mosquito venom.) Allergies cause swelling of the affected tissues, and if you eat a food or something you are allergic to, it can have very serious side effects and may result in death.

This happens because your body is so sensitive to the substance that the swelling causes your airway to close. As we have said before, the cardinal points of health begin with ABC…Airway, Breathing, and Circulation.

If you can't breathe because your airway is closed, you have lost the first two of three! This may result in severe damage to your body and may result in loss of life! If you have an allergy to any foods or drugs, you should wear a MedicAlert bracelet ***and*** you should have your allergic information on your person at all times!

The big takeaway I hope you get from this section is that some things we eat, in fact, a lot of the things we crave, are not very good for us and may make us sick after years of eating them. Keep this in mind, especially when you go for the third cup of coffee, or the dessert you really want but don't really need. The long-term effect of small things adds up after years of build-up in your system.

This can, and many times will, cause inflammation in the tissues of your body which will make your arthritis worse. You must make the best choices you can! Every choice is vital to how you feel and how your body reacts.

Osteoarthritis

Osteoarthritis (OA) is a condition where the joints of your body degenerate and become rough like RA. The difference in this type of arthritis is OA can affect people who have no genetic tendency for arthritis. It can and does affect people as a result of injuries or their lifestyle.

This means that if you abused your body playing sports as a teen, you will suffer the effects as you age. We have seen this countless times in men who play football. Men who play football for a long time have more severe problems, especially if they have suffered injury to the joints on multiple occasions.

Earl Campbell, one of the best running backs in the NFL for years, now must use a wheelchair to move around. He is one of many people who played at the highest level until his injuries kept him from playing.

You can do damage to your joints in other ways that are far less traumatic than the collisions suffered by athletes. I injured my neck snow skiing, and again when trying to act like a teenager on a cruise ship (one of those wave machines that allow you to surf threw me down so hard I had a hard time getting up). We all do things we shouldn't, and as we age we all pay the price for these oversights.

The big difference is that OA can be slowed and even stopped with the right kind of care and your dedication to the healing process. Especially when we have spinal OA, you can do exercises that stop the degeneration. If you continue your exercises at home after your in-office care is complete, you may even rebuild and regenerate your soft tissues and discs to some degree.

All forms of arthritis have variables that we may control to decrease the severity and impact the diseases have on our bodies and our lives. You must pay attention to diet and exercise with any form of arthritis. You must also make sure that you don't over-stress your body or injure yourself in a silly way when you are trying to do exercise or work that may be too difficult for your current condition.

I am constantly amazed that people (me included) don't follow the ***simple rules*** we all should know when we get hurt. So, let me restate them here in written form so you may have them when you need them…

Rules for healing when you get hurt:

1. **RICE - when you hurt yourself doing anything..Rest, Ice, Compression (use a bandage to gently apply compression to the area), and Elevation.**
2. **After an injury, do only the things you can comfortably do! If it hurts above a level of 5/10, then don't do it! You will eventually need to push yourself to make a full recovery, but people often push too hard too soon!**
3. **Start with gravity-only exercise. This means that if it hurts, even on a scale of 5/10, to move the injured joint against grav-**

ity, then only move it to the level where you just begin to feel the discomfort and NO further!

4. **Once you have the ability to move the joint against gravity and through a full range of motion, then you may begin more aggressive exercise!** I hurt my knee (basically doing nothing but jogging) and I was shocked by how slowly I had to do my rehab. I was in pretty good shape, but I literally went from being able to run five miles, to not being able to walk without being very careful. I wore a brace for over six weeks, and added exercise slowly (going up and down stairs is exercise) until I could walk several miles without pain, and then I began to walk-run!
5. **Add more difficult exercise SLOWLY! The biggest mistake most of us make (yes, me included) is trying to do too much too fast.** I have had many patients over the years who jumped from doing a little exercise to doing a lot, and then they hurt themselves so badly that they gave up! Do only the exercise that you can do...you will feel discomfort, but you should never exercise to the point of extreme or sudden pain! If you feel an unusual amount of pain while exercising, STOP!

Now that we all understand these simple rules, please understand that if you have a disease like arthritis, you will need help when you design your exercise program! Don't go to the gym and expect to be able to do all of the exercises that other people do!

You also need to understand that you can push yourself, but DON'T let anyone push you so hard that you get hurt in the process! People who have arthritis may exercise, but they must do it in the right way.

If you have any form of arthritis, you already have a tendency for joint problems. Pushing yourself to the extreme while doing exercise can put too much stress on the joints and tendons and could damage your joints beyond repair!

So when that trainer, or the little voice in your head, tells you to do "Just one more!", remember that you could do more harm than good if you do! Your arthritis can be made better by making your body stronger, but you must know your limits and never push too hard!

Juvenile Idiopathic Arthritis

By now you understand the hallmarks of this disease. It attacks the joints and the soft tissues of your body, and causes destruction of the tissues that support your frame and make you strong. Juvenile Idiopathic Arthritis (JIA) is, in my opinion, one of the worst forms of arthritis because it strikes children. As we age, most of us expect that our bodies will not be as strong as they used to be when we were young. Unfortunately, those with JIA may never have the chance to feel really strong.

JIA is a disease of the immune system. The immune system is normally the system that prevents you from getting sick. This system works by attacking any bacteria or virus that invades your body and grows inside of you, taking vital nutrients and energy that sustains you and makes you feel "normal or good."

If you have JIA, the immune system doesn't work as it should and the result is the bones, joints, muscles and cartilage are all affected. This causes an accelerated decay of the tissues and causes pain and disability.

JIA has many factors and the current research shows it has a genetic component. This means that the disease is not curable with any medicine available today. Therefore, you must make sure that you do everything you can do to lessen the symptoms of this disease and live as normal a life as you can.

One day, hopefully very soon, we will have tests that will tell you what diseases you may get throughout your life. Now there are tests available to many people that can tell you if you may pass on a gene to your child which may cause disease.

As a doctor, I feel that knowing you have a family history or tendency for disease and having children anyway is unwise. If you know your family history, and you know your child will have a high probability of being born with a disease, you are condemning the child and burdening your family with untold expenses.

That said, there are many diseases (genetically transmitted as well) that appear in families with no previous history. So, let's focus on how to make this disease less of an issue!

What we know

JIA affects all of the body tissues. You must get this form of arthritis diagnosed as quickly as possible to lessen the severity of the disease process. As in all forms of arthritis, the destruction of the tissues is the most important part of the disease. Because JIA strikes your child, you must make sure that they understand what is happening to their body, and make them understand that JIA is a disease, but it does not define who they are! (http://www.arthritis.org/conditions-treatments/disease-center/juvenile—arthritis/)

As soon as you have a proper diagnosis, you must begin the work (hard work) of making every effort to get your child's diet, exercise, medication and rest cycles managed. Don't be upset if this process takes more time than you want.

Do the best you can do every day, and understand that as your child grows you will have frequent changes to your plan of action. One day a medicine that worked great for pain may stop working, and another day your child may get suddenly worse or significantly better for no reason. This is a part of the disease process.

For that reason, you must try to keep a moderate tone when dealing with the problems related to JIA. Your child must not feel blame or the burden of the disease, if possible…just do your best!

Exercise is vitally important for anyone with arthritis, but for children with JIA, it is essential! The big takeaway for you in regard to exercise is simple…don't do any exercise that causes pain! Have your child do whatever exercise he/she can do, and ask them for feedback.

Make sure that they feel the stress of the exercise, but don't allow them to push too hard. For a normal person, I always tell them that as they age they shouldn't think about the old saying, "No pain, no gain!"

For a child with JIA, this goes double! The stress they feel from exercise should be limited to the mild burn we feel when we begin to get tired from exertion. Asking a child with bone and muscle disease to "push it hard" is asking for trouble, so don't do it. (http://www.kidsgetarthritistoo.org/living-with-ja/daily-life/staying-active/ja-exercise.php)

There may be times when your child may be in pain simply without exertion or exercise. If this is "one of those days," avoid the exercise session for the day, and do something else to get your child's mind off the pain, if possible. On these days, castor oil and a heating pad may be the only choice!

Nutrition

Nutrition may help with some of the problems associated with JIA, but it will rarely stop or correct any part of the disease. Children may suffer from the components of the disease in different ways. While some may be able to eat, or choose not to eat because they are depressed, others may use food as an outlet and may suffer with weight problems as a result of over-eating.

For this reason, the diet of your child should be closely monitored and any and all foods that aggravate arthritis should be omitted, while foods that help your child should become staples of their diet. Allergy testing may be one way to make sure your child is not exposed to foods that cause problems. Elimination diets are another, less costly way to determine if your child has a problem with a food.

Allergy testing must be done in a doctor's office. This procedure involves giving the patient a small dose of an allergen by pricking the skin and placing the allergen in the opening, or the doctor may simply drop the allergen on the skin. In order to get a more accurate result, doctors will sometimes inject the patient with the allergen. The reason these tests need to be done in a doctor's office is to prevent death from a severe allergic reaction (called anaphylaxis). (http://www.acaai.org/allergist/allergies/treatment/diagnosing-allergies/pages/allergy-testing.aspx)

After allergic substances are identified, it is vital that you avoid the food or substance! These substances can also create problems if you show a sensitivity but are not allergic. Sensitivity may also lead to problems if your child eats too much of a particular food.

We have had many patients over the years who had allergy testing done but still had problems due to food sensitivity. There have also been patients who have had problems with certain combinations of foods. This is unusual, but once these problems were identified and the diet was corrected, the suffering lessened.

The Elimination Diet can be done by anyone with a little bit of effort and dedication. What is done in this type of diet is to make a log of what types of foods your child will eat and does eat on a regular basis. Make sure you chart and log everything your child puts in his mouth, as even chewing a substance may be enough to create a reaction. After this is done, most people will begin by eliminating the foods that are the most likely to cause a reaction.

Dairy is one of the food substances that cause digestive problems in a lot of people. When you eliminate a food, you must make sure you get that food out of your diet completely! Just because your child isn't drinking milk does not mean he can eat foods which contain milk.

When you eliminate a food, take it completely out of your child's diet for at least two weeks and make sure they don't cheat, if at all possible. Many children, especially those who go to public school, have access to foods that their parents are trying to eliminate when they aren't being directly supervised. If they eat the food without telling you, how can you chart the finding that they have no problem with the food? To do this diet correctly, you must keep a very strict log, and make sure the eliminated food is truly gone from the diet for success.

When you find a food that makes a difference in how your child feels, or one that slows down his symptoms, make sure you get them to recognize how that food makes them feel when they eat it! My daughter (who is healthy, thank God) has sensitivity to milk. When she was little, we figured out through the elimination diet that milk was causing her headaches.

After we eliminated the milk, she asked me if she could have milk with her cereal one day and I told her, "Yes, dear, but if you eat milk, you'll get a headache. You need to make a decision of whether you want the milk or the headaches that come from eating the milk." She never ate milk again! (http://www.whfoods.com/genpage.php?tname=faq&dbid=30)

Medication

Typically, doctors will prescribe non-steroidal anti-inflammatory drugs (NSAIDs) first for patients with arthritis. **NSAIDs** work by inhibiting the production of cyclooxygenase (COX) which, in turn, causes inflammation, fever, and pain in the body. NSAIDs are the first line of defense for arthritis, as they are very safe drugs and very easy for most patients to use. (http://www.medicinenet.com/nonsteroidal_antiinflammatory_drugs/article.htm)

Analgesics are a class of drugs that work by blocking the pain of arthritis. These drugs have little to no effect on the swelling caused by arthritis and are drugs like Tylenol, Ultram, and other drugs that contain hydrocodone or oxycodone. These drugs will help with the pain of arthritis, but do little, if anything, to prevent further destruction in the joints.

Disease Modifying Anti-Rheumatic Drugs (DMARDs) are a class of drugs which work by slowing or stopping the attack of your immune system on the joints and soft tissues that causes arthritis. Examples of these drugs are methotrexate (Trexall) and hydroxychloroquine (Plaquenil). These drugs also help lessen the pain from arthritis.

Biologics will be prescribed by your doctor to give an added boost to the DMARDs. These drugs target different immune system triggers that cause inflammation and damage to the joints and soft tissues in arthritic patients. Etanercept (Enbrel) and infliximab (Remicade) are typical drugs that are biologics. They run interference to make sure that the DMARDs have more power in your body. Results for these drugs vary, and your doctor will need to adjust your dosage to make sure you get the best effect from the treatment.

Coritcosteroids are used to suppress swelling and also may help keep your immune system from attacking your joints. These drugs include cortisone and prednisone, and have many uses in medicine.

All drugs have side effects. Unfortunately, any drug that modifies a process in your body can have serious side effects, such as lowering your body's ability to fight off infection. You may have seen commercials for Enbrel, where they warn you about possible infections you may get after using the drug.

Your doctor will help you decide if using these drugs will give you a benefit that outweighs any risk. He/she will also give you very specific instructions on how to use the drug, and you must not discontinue these drugs without help and direction from your doctor!

You must also tell your doctor if you have any other problems. Don't assume that your cough is not a big deal when taking these medications! The warning label on these drugs is there for a reason. Failure to give vital information to your doctor will only hurt you and cause you and your loved ones to suffer needlessly.

Joint replacement is a final option for those who suffer joint destruction from arthritis. This is a surgical procedure where the doctor will literally take out part or all of the damaged joint and replace it with another artificial or harvested joint. These surgeries are getting better and better results, but with arthritis you may still need drug therapy to decrease pain and prevent other joints from being damaged.

Action Plan for Arthritis

1. Know what type of arthritis you are dealing with, and make sure you have all of the information you need regarding your disease. When you seek help from your doctor, understand all of the treatment options and the risks with each type of treatment.
2. Understand the cause of arthritis cannot be cured. This means that you must do everything you can do to lessen the effects of arthritis in your body. Make sure you keep track of how different things affect you. Many patients tell me that they feel worse when a storm is coming (they also say that their doctor doesn't believe them). Keep a written log of what causes your pain to get worse and make special notes of things that make you feel better!
3. Get rid of sugar, wheat, and milk in your diet. All of these foods can cause swelling and make your arthritis symptoms worse. However, if you do not find that getting rid of a food helps, don't eliminate it if you love it!
4. Exercise as much as you can without hurting yourself. As I age, I use less weight and do more repetition when I work out. Some people will find that just moving is an extreme workout. Don't let anyone push you beyond your limit, and be honest with yourself. You need as much exercise as your body will tolerate!
5. Make a list of all of the drugs you take (even the over-the-counter ones), and check the side effects of all the drugs, making sure to list the combined effects of the drugs. Remember that what you eat is also a factor in how well some drugs work. Don't take any new medicine without understanding how and why you are taking it. If it doesn't work for you, tell your doctor before you stop the medication. (http://www.drugs.com/drug_interactions.html)

9

Skin Disorders

Skin problems are one of the main reasons people of all ages go to the doctor. We are visual animals and, as such, we want to look as good as we can. If we don't like the way we look, we believe others will notice too. As a doctor, the main thing I'd like to communicate here is simple…your skin problem may not be as big a deal as you think it is.

…your skin problem may not be as big a deal as you think it is.

I'm not saying it isn't important, but we've all had a blemish that we think is massive, only to look in the mirror and find out it's not as big as we see it. When it comes to skin problems, we really are on overdrive most of the time! However, some skin problems can be a very big deal and can leave you with scars and can cause you great emotional pain that may last a lifetime.

There are too many pills and potions out there for almost every type of skin problem, so I'm going to focus on the most common types of skin problems and let you do the deep research if you have difficult skin. This chapter will be a guide for you and will not give you exact solutions. The real thing to understand here is to start with the basic remedies and then work your way to the more extreme remedies, if needed.

For almost everyone, skin appearance is vitally important and represents how they are seen by the outer world. If you have healthy, vibrant skin, you do look better. If you have difficult skin, like I did as a teenager, you know the pain of judgment of others who don't have a problem. I scrubbed my skin raw on many occasions trying to get rid of a blemish I thought was horrible. It can consume you and change you in very strange ways.

One of the biggest things you need to understand when it comes to your skin is to be clear on when you must go to a doctor to get help. There is a distinct difference between the care you can do for yourself and the care a doctor may give. Unlike other types of care, dermatologists are specialists and can prevent you from doing more damage when you try using chemicals or scrubs, which can cause scarring if used improperly.

There are a lot of different types of skin problems, and there are many different books and resources that you could use to determine what type of care may help your specific problem. For the purposes of this chapter, we will only focus on the top skin problems that cause people to see the doctor.

Your skin is the biggest organ of your body and protects you from infection and dehydration.

Your skin is the biggest organ of your body and protects you from infection and dehydration. You must protect your skin and make sure that you don't do something that happens very easily…spread an infection or allergy from one part of your body to another part by scratching the affected area. When you get an area of infection or irritation on your skin and you scratch that area, you may transfer the thing that causes the problem on your fingertips or under your fingernails.

I have had many patients come in with this problem and claim that they couldn't have done this because they wash and clean their hands. The problem is, they can't really clean their fingers and nails enough.

Even after washing, the irritant may still pass from one place to another on your skin or under your nails when you touch or scratch the affected area and then touch your skin again. This is called auto-infection. (http://medical-dictionary.thefreedictionary.com/autoinfection)

We had a patient who had been to several doctors for a difficult skin problem. She showed me her arms and she had a rash from her wrists to above her elbows on both sides. From our visit I was able to determine that she got some sort of allergen on her skin and literally scratched it up her own arms (called auto-infection).

We had to treat her for the rash and the infection she caused from scratching. The big problem was that her skin was so damaged, she needed to use less medication to get her skin to heal. We used a combination of antibiotics to treat her infected skin and castor oil to soothe her skin and prevent further problems.

After several weeks her skin was healing nicely! We used a very simple and inexpensive remedy to fix a problem that had gotten out of hand, and the patient was thrilled. That's what I call a win-win!

Acne

Acne is the most common reason people go to the doctor. As I said before, most of us suffer with acne in our youth. As our bodies change during puberty, we secrete hormones that literally change every part of our body. One of the most embarrassing changes for me as a youth was the change that caused my skin to break out.

As we grow into young adulthood, our body secretes androgens (male and female hormones) which help us to mature. Unfortunately, hormones cause the skin to change from the fine, smooth skin we have as babies, into the rougher skin we all have as adults. This change also affects the pores of the skin and causes the pores of the skin to get clogged. When the clogged pore gets infected or blocked, we may get blackheads, whiteheads, or cysts.

...hormones cause the skin to change from the fine, smooth skin we have as babies, into the rougher skin we all have as adults.

Blackheads are a clogged pore that has a darker color plug in the pore. The problem is blackheads stop the oil produced in the pore from coming out and this backup makes the pore and the skin around it sensitive. As the oil builds up you may develop a bump, and in bad cases you can develop an infection of your skin behind this blocked pore.

Whiteheads for me were even worse than the blackheads. Whiteheads develop when the pore gets blocked, but this block is a bit deeper in the pore and the body reacts by producing pus and a visible infection with redness and swelling that appears around the blocked pore. This is the typical "zit" we all hate!

There is one other type of acne, called cystic acne, which is the worst type, in my opinion. In this type of acne, the blocked pore is infected at a deeper level and a cyst, or pocket of infection, develops deep in the skin layers. This cyst can damage the skin at a level that leaves a scar or a "pock mark." (http://www.medicinenet.com/acne/article.htm)

If you have acne, you probably don't care which type of blemish you have, you simply want the blemishes gone! The best news is there is a lot of great help out there, and it seems to be getting better every day! But you need to choose your sources wisely, and don't get caught up in any of the online scams that will cost you money and leave you with damaged skin and an empty wallet.

Normal acne requires several types of attention to prevent skin infection and spreading of the disease.

1. As bad as it sounds, don't pick at the zits! I have literally seen medical doctors attack a blemish on their own face and squeeze it, only to criticize themselves afterwards for doing what they tell others to avoid! The problem with this is it can (and often will) drive the infection deeper into the skin, producing more damage than if left alone.
2. When you get acne, you must take care to keep your hands and your face clean. Your hands are rarely, if ever, clean enough. Washing your hands may help keep your skin and face clean when you touch yourself. Use a gentle cleaner for your face so you don't over-dry your skin.
3. Get yourself tested for food allergies and sensitivities. Your acne may be aggravated by your diet, especially cow's milk, and diets that are high in foods containing sugar or foods that easily convert to sugar (high glycemic diets). I noticed a great improvement in my skin when I eliminated gluten from my diet. Much of the more recent research shows that other foods (like chocolate) do not directly affect your acne. (http://www.ncbi.nlm.nih.gov/pubmed/20361171)
4. Be careful when wearing hats or other things that press against your skin. The pressure from a hat, especially a hard hat, can cause a flare-up of acne. I had a hard time with acne in high

school during football season from the helmet pressing against my face!

5. When your acne becomes bad and you have done everything you can, you need to go see the doctor. We all hate to go to the doctor, but there are times when you need professional help! Doctors can give you antibiotics to help your body deal with the infections acne causes, and this can help your body recover and prevent scarring of your skin. I have had personal experience with this, and I felt like a bit of a failure during my visit, but was assured that drugs were needed to prevent more aggressive therapy.

Drugs for acne

Drugs should be a last line of defense when dealing with acne. However, don't let your acne get too far out of control before you seek care! You can always stop taking the drugs, but the only sure way to rid your face of the scars from acne is with plastic surgery.

Doctors will use creams or gels first to try to dry up the blemishes. These creams are fairly standard through the industry and they do one thing…they dry up the oil that causes your pores to get clogged. The problem with these creams is they dry up everything else as well, so you may get very dry skin that flakes as a result of using them.

The most common type of cream you use on your skin will say "noncomedogenic" on the label.

The most common type of cream you use on your skin will say "noncomedogenic" on the label. This means the cream prevents the formation of the comedone or pimple in your skin pores. It is very important to make the proper choice of cream for your skin type.

Those that have a drying agent (benzoyl peroxide or salicylic acid) ingredient are going to dry more than other non-alcohol creams and can be very irritating. Today there are a lot of different strengths and combinations of ingredients available over the counter, so make sure you buy different types when you change.

If you have already tried as much as you feel is reasonable to rid your skin of the acne, it's time for a change to stronger medications. For this you will need to go to the dermatologist, who specializes in skin conditions. Many times we have seen patients in our office who want us to prescribe something for themselves or their child who has acne. I always ask them to go to the specialist!

Simply put, a lot of skin conditions and diseases look alike. You will probably be much happier and get the right type of treatment from an expert who specializes in skin conditions than from another type of doctor.

Dermatologists will most likely start with tretinoin cream. As mentioned before, this cream will dry up your skin and you may find it too irritating. There are other creams that don't dry as much, or that combine drying agents with antibiotics to give you an option for your skin problem. Adapalene is a topical medicine that works well for some people, but it needs to be used for at least 12 weeks to get the full effect. (http://www.mayoclinic.com/health/drug-information/DR600039/DSECTION=before-using)

Other medications include azelaic acid, antibiotics such as erythromycin or clindamycin, combined with sodium sulfacetamide. These products work by breaking down the blocked skin pore and treating the infection with a small amount of antibiotic contained in the cream. You need to be careful in the sun when you use these products, and you need to read all of the information about foods that may interact with the medicine, or which may cause a side effect during use.

Benzamycin and Benzaclin are combinations of benzoyl peroxide and an antibiotic, but are prescription only drugs. Strictly speaking, gel medications are typically more drying than creams. If you have a skin problem, you need to decide what kind of delivery system you will use. Lotions and scrubs may be used together, but make sure to consult your doctor for instructions if you plan to use anything else with your prescribed medication! You could damage your skin by using too much medicine, or create a reaction by using products that have a bad interaction.

You also need to be aware that your skin is being affected by all of the medicine you take, combined with foods, vitamins, and anything you might put on your skin. You will more than likely be more sensitive to the sun. This means you will burn your skin more easily, and you may even need to avoid sun exposure!

The most important thing for you to do is to be aware that these problems may exist and avoid damaging your skin. These sensitivities will go away (for most people) after the medication has cleared from your system.

Women may find significant help from acne by using hormones. It has long been known that women seem to get better if they use hormone therapy to stop breakouts. Oral birth control pills are the number one choice for this type of therapy, but your doctor may use a testosterone blocker as well.

The contraceptives that work the best for women who use them are Ortho Tri-Cyclen, Estrostep, and Yaz, but all contraceptive pills have a similar effect. The reason this happens is the hormones cause the ovaries and adrenal glands in a woman's body to produce less testosterone. Less testosterone, DHT, and androgens equals fewer acne blemishes. (http://www.acne.org/women-and-acne.html#birth-control)

Action plan for Acne

1. Make sure you understand what you can do and must do to prevent your skin from breaking out. Adjust your diet; remove all foods you may be sensitive to from your diet. Make sure you avoid sugars and greasy or fried foods.
2. Wash your skin and your hands frequently, but not enough to create skin sensitivity or abrasions from the washing or scrubbing.
3. Use over-the-counter products containing benzoyl peroxide (2.5%) or salicylic acid to dry up the acne and prevent new breakouts. Use these products carefully, and make sure to report any unwanted effects to your doctor. Be careful with any medication to avoid sun exposure and to avoid foods that interact with any medication.
4. Make sure you understand when you need professional help from a qualified doctor for your acne. You should see a doctor if you have acne that does not respond to your home treatments, and if you are concerned that you may get permanent scarring from your acne, or you have deep cystic acne that stops you or prevents you from wanted social activities.
5. Once you make the decision to visit your doctor, go with specific goals in mind. Let your doctor know what you want and stay committed to the plan. Do everything he/she prescribes for you, and make sure you know when to move to the next treatment. Isotretinoin or Accutane is usually a last resort drug and should be used only if you understand ***all of the risks!***

Eczema

Eczema is a skin condition that is diagnosed by doctors when you have a dry skin problem that is itchy and may flake. From the research, all types of eczemaand there are five types (atopic dermatitis, contact dermatitis, seborrheic dermatitis, dyshidrotic eczema, and nummular eczema) — have the same pattern. There are a ton of creams and lotions out there to treat eczema. Some have benefits, and others are useless. We recommend several steps that work fairly well for eczema patients.

Drugs and treatments - There are mainly two ways your doctor will treat eczema, with topical steroids and topical immunomodulators. The goal of these drugs is to stop the swelling of thc tissucs and to prevent further breakdown of the skin. You will use the topical steroids on your skin to prevent swelling in the affected area. Immunomodulators are drugs that work by suppressing your body's immune system and this prevents inflammation or swelling. These have some really awful side effects, and you should make sure you understand all of the risks of use before beginning treatment with this class of drug. (http://www.webmd.com/drugs/drug-22383-Elidel+Top.aspx?drgid=22383&drugname=Elidel+Top)

ACTION PLAN FOR ECZEMA

1. Define the type of eczema you have. The more you know about your type, the better your chances will be of getting results without wasting time and money.
2. Take care of your skin daily. Wear softer clothes that don't scratch or irritate your skin, and use lotions or creams to soothe your skin. Don't take baths or showers that are too hot, or use soaps that irritate, as these will cause more problems for your skin.
3. Alter your diet, if necessary. Many people with eczema find that eliminating dairy and grain from their diet helps their skin. You may also find that getting rid of animals and carpets in your environment will also help, because many people are allergic or sensitive to pet dander or synthetic fibers in carpet.
4. Avoid sudden changes in temperature, and use a humidifier in the winter to prevent additional drying of your skin.
5. As simple as it sounds, don't scratch your skin — and trim the nails of children with eczema to prevent infections or skin breakdown from scratching.

Psoriasis

This condition is another skin condition that is the result of immune system disease. The skin in this disease produces too quickly, and the result is patches of raised, red, scaly or silvery skin that may bleed (plaques). These raised areas can itch and burn, and the plaques may flake and cause you to try to cover up the area. There are options for care when you suffer with psoriasis. The main source of treatment focuses on the over-production of proteins called tumor necrosis factors (TNFs) that actually cause the over-production of skin.

Drug therapy for psoriasis slows the over-production of skin cells and smooths the skin. There are other types of treatments, such as phototherapy (light therapy) or topical medications, which help to smooth the skin. These treatments all will focus on slowing down how fast your body makes new skin cells, which is the reason the plaques build up.

Action Plan for Psoriasis

1. Again, you need to identify what type of psoriasis you have to make sure you get the right type of care. There are many types of psoriasis; your diagnosis needs to be made by a ***doctor who specializes in dermatology!***
2. Take daily baths to remove the excess skin, use moisturizers, cover the plaqued areas of skin at night, and make sure you avoid triggers and expose your skin to small amounts of sunlight. Try topical over-the-counter medications first. Always stop any medication that causes a rash or itching on any part of your body. (https://www.psoriasis.org/sublearn03_mild_otc)
3. You will also want to avoid drinking alcohol and you must eat a healthy diet to lessen your symptoms. You may also want to consider adding aloe vera and fish oil to your diet to help with the inflammation of your skin. We have patients who report that a gluten-free diet helps!
4. If you don't get relief from your psoriasis with creams and moisturizers, or over-the-counter medications that contain steroids and anti-itch ingredients, then move on to prescription medications recommended by a dermatologist.
5. Last, you will need a dermatologist who may prescribe phototherapy or laser treatment and then ingested or injected medications to help your symptoms. Retinoids, methotrexate, cyclosporine, hydroxyurea, and immunomodulators are used, and all have different side effects you must be aware of to lessen the chance of complications from their use. (http://www.mayoclinic.com/health/psoriasis/DS00193/DSECTION=treatments-and-drugs)

Skin Cancer

Skin cancers are one of the most dangerous skin diseases. There are basically two different types of skin cancers...melanoma or non-melanoma cancers. Skin cancer is also the most common form of cancer. All skin problems should be documented by using a simple A-B-C-D-E system.

A is for asymmetry. When you look at a spot on your body, you will see that one-half of the spot is unusually shaped when compared to the other half. This signals that the cells of the mole or birthmark have changed and ***you need to get a doctor's opinion of the lesion.*** Any change in an area of your skin that looks uneven, especially if the spot looked even before, could be a very big deal.

B stands for border. When you look at the outer edges of a spot or birthmark, has the outer edge or border changed in its normal appearance? If the edges look irregular, notched or blurred, and especially if this was not the case before, the border of the spot has changed!

C represents the color of the skin in the area. If a mole changes from brown to black, or if there are other colors that appear like blue, red, pink or white, it is a bad sign that requires an examination by a dermatologist. You also need to pay attention if the hair growing in a spot changes color as well.

D is for diameter, or the distance across the spot. If the spot is six millimeters across (about the size of an average pencil eraser), then you need to have it examined by your doctor. For these problems, it will be best for you to seek the advice of a qualified dermatologist. I have had many patients over the years that have asked me what a spot is, or if they should be worried about a change in a spot. I always refer them to a dermatologist! They simply know better than I if a spot is just a spot, or if it needs to be examined more thoroughly.

E is for evolving or elevation. If a mole or a spot that was flat is no longer flat, or if a spot continues to change as you check it over time, then you need help! Help means go to the dermatologist.

You will also need to be careful if you have an open spot or wound that doesn't heal or bleeds easily, a mole or spot that has color that spreads to the surrounding skin, redness or swelling around a mole, or if you begin to itch or have a change in sensation. (http://www.cancer.org/cancer/skincancer-melanoma/detailedguide/melanoma-skin-cancer-detection)

After the doctor sees you for a skin lesion, he will decide if the lesion needs to be sampled for examination. This may be done by scraping the skin, cutting the skin, or getting a full thickness sample of the spot by doing a punch biopsy. He will then send the sample to a lab that will check the cells and type them to see if there is cancer in the sampled tissue. If your doctor tells you that there are cancer cells in the sample, you need to do what he tells you to do!

I had a spot on my body that looked rough, uneven, and was in a very delicate place. I went to one doctor who specialized in that area for men, and he told me I had a cancer that needed to be removed immediately. My wife and I were freaked out and scared to death, because this guy wanted to schedule surgery the next day.

I called another doctor who told me to go to a dermatologist. Not wanting the surgery, and hoping for a better diagnosis, I made the appointment. Two minutes into the exam, the dermatologist took tweezers, removed the spot and announced it was a scab!

Cancer can be deadly, but skin cancer is usually treatable. Make sure your diagnosis is correct and don't be afraid. Waiting only prolongs your suffering and can make a simple problem a surgical problem.

Action Plan for Skin Cancer

1. Avoid the sun during the mid-day and wear protective clothing or sun-screen to lessen your exposure.
2. Make sure you know when you are using medications that may make your skin more sensitive to the sun (common photo-toxic drugs are the tetracycline family, NSAIDs [non-steroidal anti-inflammatory drugs such as ibuprofen], and amiodarone, a heart medication. (http://www.webmd.com/skin-problems-and-treatments/sun-sensitizing-drugs)
3. Check your skin regularly and have someone else check areas you cannot see. Report directly to your doctor any changes you see as soon as you see changes in the area, or if you experience any of the problems listed above.
4. The earlier you go to the doctor, the less surgery you are likely to need! Small lesions don't usually require surgery, so if you think a spot may be cancerous, don't delay your care, ***it won't go away on its own!***
5. If you get bad news, follow your doctor's recommendations exactly! There are a lot of times I would tell you to try other ways to heal your body, but when it comes to cancer (or something that might be), I will tell you to please get professional advice and help!

Some of the things you may like to try involve keeping your treatments simple. If your skin is weeping or oily, try drying it gently. If your skin is dry, add an oil or lotion that works well for you. We always ask our patients to try castor oil first. It is inexpensive and it works for most conditions without any problems.

10
Cholesterol Problems

Cholesterol is a natural substance that occurs in your body and is also a result of normal digestion. Some of the cholesterol in your body is actually involved in vital processes and everyone who is alive has cholesterol. You need to understand there are two different types of cholesterol and what makes the levels of each type go up or down. Everyone who cares seems to be focused on cholesterol numbers and how to keep the "bad" number down.

"Good cholesterol" is the cholesterol called HDL, or a high density lipoprotein (think "H" for healthy). This type of cholesterol actually is better for you if the number is higher. This type of cholesterol is supposedly helpful in your body and may help prevent heart attacks. The truth is, no one really knows if this is true yet! Don't buy into the hype, especially if you are trying to get higher HDL with drugs. The results so far are not good! (http://pjmedia.com/blog/does-a-high-level-of-good-cholesterol-really-help-prevent-heart-attacks/2/)

"Bad cholesterol" is the term used for LDL, or low-density lipoprotein (think "L" for lousy). This type of cholesterol is known to have a part in heart-related problems, but there are countries in the world where most people have high LDL levels with little increases in the rate of heart disease. (http://life.gaiam.com/article/why-cholesterol-may-not-be-cause-heart-disease)

We have been educated by the media and our doctors that cholesterol is a major contributor to heart disease. We believe doctors because of their education, and our trust comes from their ability to correctly help us get better when we are ill. The dirty little secret in medicine is…most doctors are taught how to treat disease. This means they (we) have a standard formula they follow when a patient presents with a particular health challenge.

For cholesterol, we (most of us) rely on the information we were given regarding studies that were done by the pharmaceutical companies when the drug was developed. These studies showed that LDL cholesterol was a big problem that caused heart disease and the solution was to use drugs to lower the "bad cholesterol." The drugs used for this purpose are called statins.

Statins are drugs like Lipitor and Zocor which lower the LDL in your blood. Statins work in a very specific way. According to research, statins block an enzyme called HMG-CoA reductase, which controls cholesterol production in the liver. Statins replace the HMG-CoA that exists in the liver, which slows down the cholesterol production process. Additional enzymes in the liver cells sense that cholesterol production has decreased and respond by creating a protein that leads to an increase in the production of LDL (low density lipoprotein, or "bad" cholesterol) receptors. This may help lower LDL even further.

The hope is that statins will cause new connections of receptors in the liver which will help your body digest LDL and VLDL (very low density lipoprotein) in the liver. This process helps lower

LDL that is dangerous because it clogs the blood vessels in your body and this may cause a heart attack or a stroke. Almost all statins work in this way, but it is also important to exercise to reduce your cholesterol. (http://www.medicalnewstoday.com/articles/8274.php)

Now, here is where the rubber meets the road…there is now proof that statins cause damage to your liver and other organs in your body! Your eyes actually use cholesterol for nutrition, and research shows that statin use may actually speed up the development of cataracts in your eyes. Research also shows that statins affect the muscles in your body and could cause muscle cells to break down in some people.

I have a friend who was diagnosed with high cholesterol (hypercholesterolemia) by his MD. He began taking statins to lower his LDL and the numbers looked good on his next blood test. Then he began to feel bad. He called me and asked what I thought might be wrong. We went through his history and I told him that one of the more common side effects of statins was muscle soreness. He told me that his pain was more than just soreness, but he changed his diet, and stopped the statins with his doctor's help. Years later, he is sure that the statins were the problem!

This is an example of why you must develop an expert plan of what your body needs. If you have the proper information, you would know that cholesterol is mainly made inside your body! Even though you can lower your cholesterol by eating right, studies show that over 60% of the cholesterol reported on a blood test is made by your body. This means that some people will never get their numbers down because they have genetically-driven high cholesterol! (http://www.medicalnewstoday.com/articles/8274.php)

Action Plan for High Cholesterol

1. The first step to getting your cholesterol under control is recognizing that you may have a problem and getting your blood tested. Then, know your cholesterol numbers and set a realistic goal of where you want to be!
2. Clean up your diet. Eat less red meat, way less fried food, more fish and chicken, and as many (raw) veggies as you can! These steps alone will help you lower your LDL.
3. Exercise every day if you can. You don't need to turn yourself into a gym rat (although it wouldn't hurt), but get about thirty minutes of exercise per day and make sure you don't overdo!
4. If you smoke, STOP! Smoking and being overweight are the one-two punch to your heart, and high cholesterol will add fuel to the fire. If you want to try some natural products which seem to help, try red rice yeast, which is a natural source of statins.
5. If you try everything above and your cholesterol is still out of range, you probably have genetic factors which drive your cholesterol. This may mean you may need to resort to medication to get your numbers down. Read the research and make sure you understand the risks of any medicine you use before taking the medicine!

11

Anxiety and Mental Problems

Anxiety is a term that can be used to describe a number of different feelings. When these feelings cause a wanted or good response in the person who feels them, the anxiety can be termed a "good event." However, many times those who suffer from anxiety disorders feel **almost any event** is a "bad event" and, as a result, the term anxiety is generally used as a negative or "bad event" for most people.

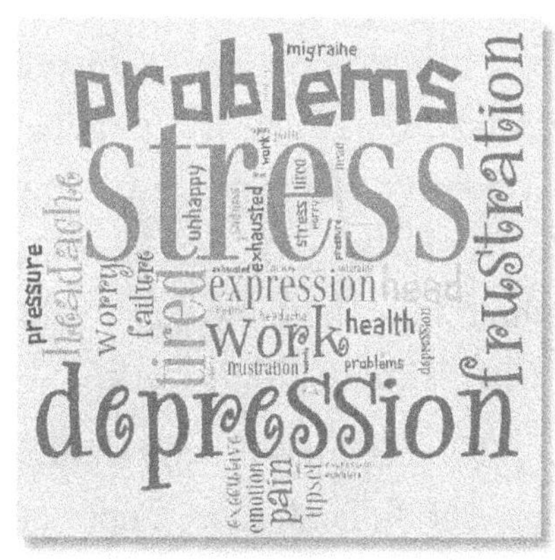

The real problem with any of the anxiety or mental disorders we encounter is the energy associated with the person who is affected. There are numerous stories of people (even twins) who had very nearly the same problem or event in their life, but the event caused a different outcome in each person. What this shows is that ***you are ultimately in control of your outcome (anxiety)!***

If you have any doubt that this statement is true, just go to your local airport and watch the people (if you are able). Everyone in an airport who is traveling is subject to very nearly the same experience, but not everyone experiences the airport travel event in the same way. Some people are unaffected by the experience, some have different levels of anxiety, and others lose control!

If you have anxiety you may experience worry, fear, nervousness, or apprehension when you are in a specific place or situation. The feelings may be normal, but your reaction to these feelings may be debilitating. So the real question is, how do you manage these episodes so they don't ruin your day?

Again, there are a lot of different treatments for anxiety. You could spend hours of your day looking on the Internet to decide what you could do to help with your symptoms. Make sure you know what you hope to accomplish before you start searching for answers. Sit down and write out what your anxiety feels like and be specific about what you want to do. If you have this information, you can then go after a treatment that is likely to help.

As with any disease, anxiety has triggers that you may be able to control. If you try to stop your anxiety by using a method and it doesn't work, it doesn't mean that this technique doesn't work! Many times we have seen patients that tell us they have tried something to make their lives better and they report (rather vigorously) that it simply didn't work.

The person is always right. When we look objectively at what the patient did and, more important ***when they did it,*** we find that they were almost doomed to fail. If you are already overloaded with too much stress, trying to remove a trigger probably won't work!

This is why you may need some help. Your body and, more important, your brain, can only handle so much at one time. If you were able to lift 20 pounds and suddenly were required to lift 100 pounds, you would fail unless you used a tool to help you lift the weight. The same logic applies to your brain and how you handle stress and triggers for anxiety.

The best way to handle anxiety and anxiety disorders is to find out what you are responding to, and then develop a strategy that you can use to lessen the stress. Many times you will need help to do this. Asking someone you already know may not work because they already have an idea about you. Look for help from an objective, qualified person who has already helped others with the same problem.

General Anxiety Triggers

Anxiety can be triggered from a host of different things, so this list is by no means meant to be complete. If you see your trigger here, great! If you don't, please don't assume that you have a bigger problem, or that you were intentionally left out. Everyone can have different triggers for stress and anxiety!

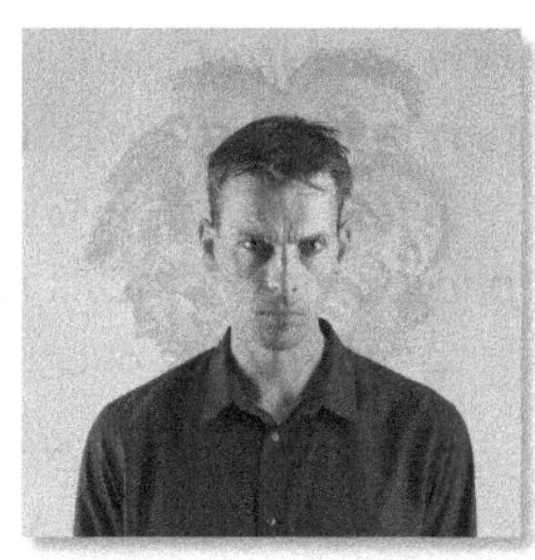

Some of the most common triggers are environmental, medical (drugs), substance use or abuse, brain function, and genetic factors. Looking at each type of trigger will not help you unless you identify ***how the trigger affects you.*** So, before you go any further, take a minute and write down the following:

1. How do I feel when I feel anxious? Are there any physical signs or symptoms of my anxiety?
2. Does my anxiety have a specific time or does it occur in a specific situation?
3. How does this affect me specifically? Do I really want a life with-

out this stress? (If the answer to this question is "No," then you may need professional help to deal with the issue.)

One of the biggest things we see in our practice when people are stressed is a sense of over-whelm. One of the most common things we hear is, "I don't know what to do. I should have some idea, shouldn't I?" The truth is, we are all much harder on ourselves than we should be. There are times in everyone's life when we all feel "lost."

Negative self-talk can have a profoundly damaging effect on anyone. Let go of the things you have little or no control of when it comes to life choices. It will save you hundreds of hours of grief!

...a study revealed that over 80% of what most people worry about is useless.

I have read many things about how to manage stress and worry, but the most helpful one I read was simple…it said that a study revealed that over 80% of what most people worry about is useless. This is because they have absolutely no control over these things! (http://www.pickthebrain.com/blog/stop-worrying/)

After reading this and other articles on worry and stress, I decided that I am a bit lazy. I figured out that if I were able to play any sport or be right about anything over 80% of the time, most people would think I was brilliant. So I decided that I would quit worrying about most things that upset me. Now, I realize that I don't do this with as much success as I had hoped, but even when I am wrong, I'm only wrong 20% of the time! That's a great result from being lazy!

If this seems a bit silly, consider that people find strange comfort from many things. You may worry about things that other people consider to be unimportant. The strange truth is, both sides of this argument have an equal claim to the truth when it comes to stress and anxiety.

Please consider the fact that something you perceive to be stressful could be pleasurable to another person. It really comes down to how you react to a situation or stressful event. If you are a bit like me, ask yourself the following, “Is this something I can really control or change?” If not, give it only the minimum amount of thought or energy you want to give it.

One thing I am sure of is the following...***you must develop a strategy that works for you!*** This is vital to your success. If you don’t follow through with this important point, you may fail in your desire to feel less stress and have a better life!

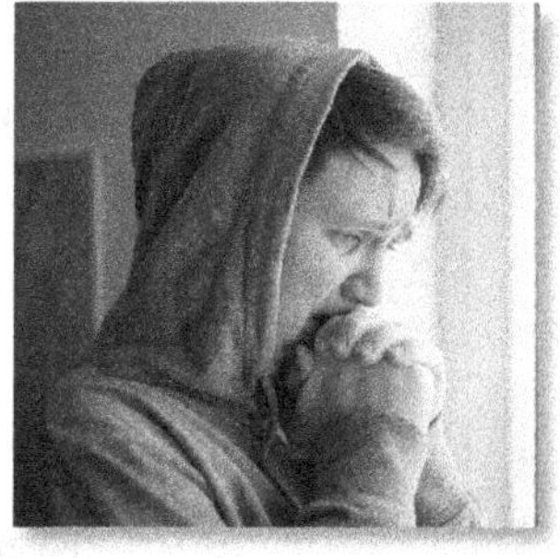

If you get to a point that creates stress or anxiety and you don’t have a strategy that works well for you, you will most likely fall back into your old reaction and your problems will continue to affect you. To make a change that works for you, you must be certain that you can change your reaction to the event.

One big takeaway you need to understand is...treat your anxiety before it becomes a bigger problem! Even mild anxiety needs to be treated, because most people who suffer from anxiety disorder start with mild anxiety that has worsened. If you start early and learn the steps you can take to help stop or lessen your anxiety, you may not need drug therapy in the future! (http://www.calmclinic.com/anxiety/types/mild-anxiety)

Understanding what triggers do to you, and how you can short-circuit those triggers, is the first step to managing anxiety and stress! Start the process by determining if you can stop anxiety with self-directed treatment. Knowing what triggers your anxiety reaction is the first step.

If you determine that you cannot stop your reaction to stress by yourself, it's time to get some help from a professional. There are many types of counselors and all of them work for someone. Whenever I need help, I ask others (professional and ordinary folks). Sometimes, this does several things that I find very helpful…

1. Professionals will tell me honestly if they have ever had a similar problem. If they did, they may have a lot of useful ideas! Take only what you think may help you! Don't take the advice of another person who has anxiety as an expert in treatment…their experience and problem is probably very different from yours!
2. If you share your problem with the person/s who is/are the ***cause of some of your stress,*** they may be willing to help you! Now you have real help with your problem! The one/s causing stress is/are now willing to help you by changing their input. This happens more often than you may think! (But, do not assume that people at work or home will react to your problem in a predictable way!)
3. When I get good input from someone, they will usually follow up with me in the future. This helps me by validating my effort in dealing with the problem and I always thank them for their help (even if their actions didn't help at all).

I decided one year that I was going to get in shape and run in a half-marathon with my wife. Everything was going well until I ran five miles on one day and three the next day. Then, my left knee swelled up and I injured it again a week later. I couldn't walk without pain, and everyone I knew gave me advice. Then a gentleman who had done the same thing to his knee told me that my fear of surgery was unfounded. He told me his surgery was easy and he recovered completely!

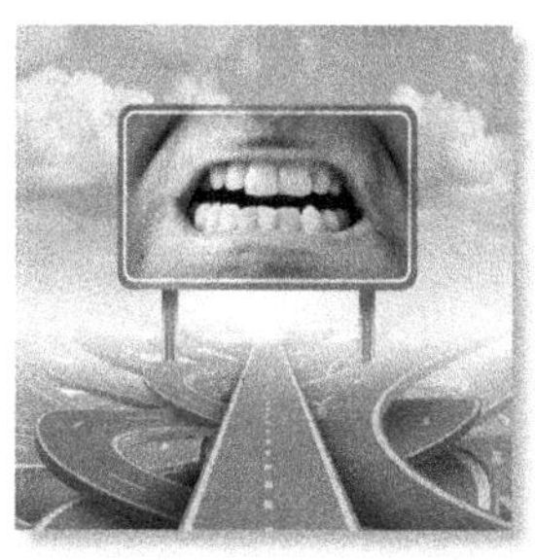

The next week I got an MRI that showed my knee needed surgery. I consulted two doctors and scheduled the surgery within two weeks. Immediately after the surgery, I was able to walk for the first time in two months without pain! I made a complete recovery and was able to enjoy life again with no pain! None of the things I feared came to pass! This is an example of how fear and anxiety can block you (or me) from a needed act!

Action Plan for Anxiety

1. The first step to treating yourself is to find out how anxiety affects you! A short pencil is better than a long memory, so write your feelings and thoughts down! Remember how anxiety affects you, what you feel, who is involved in your stress, and when you feel it. Then write down what you want from your life and how this problem stops you from getting it!
2. If you are going to try to treat yourself first (which I suggest), ask others if they have the same problems and feelings and get some input about how to start. Get simple, honest advice and don't share with anyone who may not care about you or who isn't interested in your success!
3. Learn how to help yourself. ***Do not allow negative self-talk to exist or continue!*** I have caught myself thousands of times speaking hatefully to me! When this happens, start over and see if you can find a way to change the way you talk to yourself. Focus on the things you are good at, and work to improve your strengths! You may still have some weaknesses, but don't focus on them as much! There are many millionaire athletes who stink at one part of a game, but they are millionaires because their strengths outshine their weaknesses.
4. Take time for you! Meditate, exercise, rest, and do everything you can to stop yourself from getting too stressed out. Remember that stress can be used as a motivator, and use it for that purpose only. You are in control of everything in your life until you give your control away!
5. If you try everything, or think you may need help to overcome your anxiety, get help! The longer you wait to treat your anxiety,

the harder it is to get it under control. Learn your options before going to the doctor or therapist, and make wise choices about your care. (http://www.medicalnewstoday.com/info/anxiety/anxiety-treatments)

Mental Problems

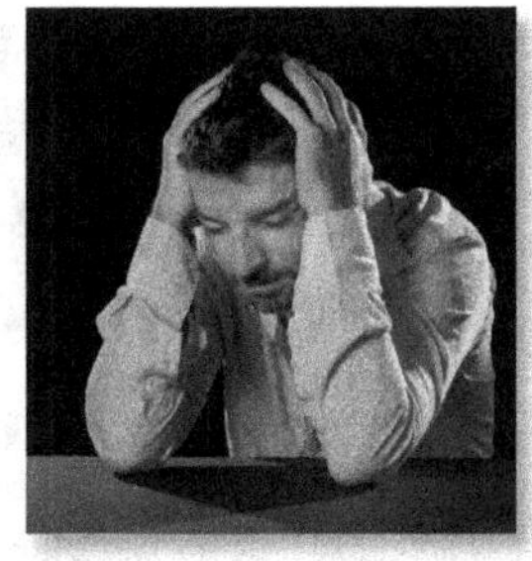

Mental problems cover a wide range of conditions. There are really too many to write about individually unless you want this book to be about two hundred pages longer, in which case you need another book! So for ease of use, I will go over the most common mental problems and not the ones that really require immediate medical attention.

Mood Disorders - Mood disorders are emotions that are sustained, or that continue when the person doesn't want them to continue. These types of disorders are very commonly diagnosed, but they may be difficult to diagnose and treat. These disorders include bipolar disorder, major depressive disorder, and dysthymic disorder.

If you have major depression, you feel sad, hopeless and worthless. Your feelings are difficult to control, and you will usually feel this way for most of your life. You may feel constantly tired or fatigued, suffer from a lack of focus, and have changes in your appetite, and you may suffer with suicidal thoughts. This makes it very difficult for you to function on a day-to-day basis and, for most people, this disease ***requires professional assistance!*** (http://www.mayoclinic.com/health/depression/DS00175/DSECTION=treatments-and-drugs)

The thing you need to understand about depression is the real effect it has on your brain. Although there is no known cause that has been identified, the factors that contribute to this disease are genetics, hormones, brain chemistry, life events and childhood trauma. The brain and its chemistry can alter the way you see the world, and this affects the way you feel about everything.

Personality Disorders - Personality disorders include antisocial behaviors, avoidant behaviors, and borderline personality disorder.

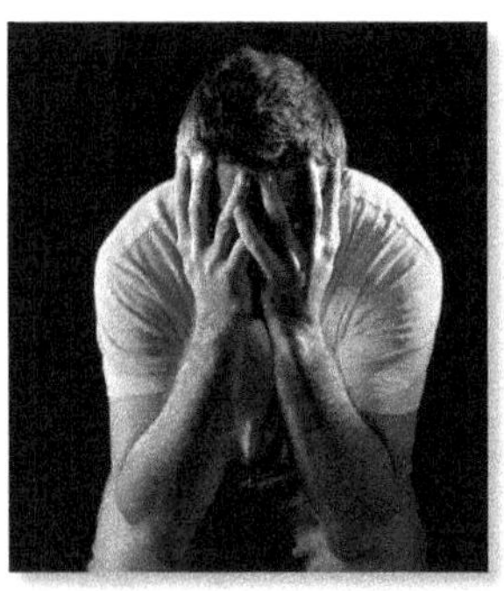

Antisocial disorder describes people who do not follow the rules of society and who have little or no regard for others or their feelings. These people may exhibit criminal behavior and have little regard for the consequences of criminal acts. These disorders may cause the person to be unaware that they need treatment or to even accept treatment when confronted. They will often need help by a loved one or family member and may need lifetime care. Drug treatment may not work for those who have antisocial disorders. (http://www.mayoclinic.org/diseases-conditions/antisocial-personality-disorder/basics/treatment/con-20027920)

Avoidant personality disorder is a disorder of people who are afraid of criticism and may be over-controlled. Their anxiety stops them from getting involved with others and they have a hard time starting and staying in relationships. Researchers think genetics and environmental causes may contribute to the development of this disorder, but little is known about the actual cause. (http://www.healthline.com/health/avoidant-personality-disorder)

A person with borderline personality disorder will be unstable and will act without thinking, or may threaten to harm or kill himself. He or she will have problems with abandonment and they often will have problems maintaining a stable relationship. As with the other types of personality disorders, the causes seem to stem from family, genetic, and social factors, which all play a part in the development of the disorder. (http://www.nlm.nih.gov/medlineplus/ency/article/000935.htm)

As a health care professional, I have a hard time understanding why people with mental challenges have a hard time getting health care. This group is constantly under pressure, and is in need of help almost daily. This is one area of your health that cannot be left alone or ignored. If you or someone you know has moderate to severe mental health issues, PLEASE get professional help! These problems typically get worse without treatment.

Action Plan for Mental Problems

1. Determine which type of problems you are dealing with and move ***quickly*** to get the help necessary for the person you love or yourself. ***Never attempt to treat yourself!*** Many times people are wrong about the type of mental problem/s, and they diagnose themselves wrong!
2. Remember exercise and diet are factors that affect everything. Get the best food you can afford, and exercise regularly to help manage the problem/s. Understand that mental health is critical to your well-being, and care may be a lifetime event.
3. A psychologist and a psychiatrist do similar things, but ***are not the same!*** Both may refer you to another type of professional to help the problem, but the psychiatrist may be better suited to your needs if you need medication to manage the symptoms of your disease. Make your choice for care and follow the recommendations of your care-giver exactly for the best results!
4. Family members should be included in therapy, if at all possible. You will need a strong support structure for your therapy to succeed. This means you may need to exclude those people close to you who are not committed to your health and well-being. Look at tendencies in those who may have these problems; family problems and abuse may lead to mental problems in adulthood.
5. Never change or stop your therapy without the direction and consent of your chosen medical provider. The results could be disastrous and/or dangerous.

12

Neurologic Problems

According to current research, there are over 600 different neurological disorders that have been defined or diagnosed. We will review the most common reasons people go to the neurologist and apologize in advance to you if your problem is missed in this book. It would be too hard to go over every type of problem, and we couldn't possibly do a good job if we tried. (http://www.nlm.nih.gov/medlineplus/neurologicdiseases.html or http://www.neurological.org.nz/disorders)

Headaches are the main reason people wind up in a neurologist's office. We have information on headaches that has already been written in another area of this book. Please make sure that you know the main types of headaches, what can cause them, and which type of headache you think you have before your visit.

Make sure you tell the doctor what you have done, what works and doesn't work, and how long you have been suffering. Keep a list of any triggers that may start a headache and let your doctor and his team help you design a treatment plan that will help you live headache-free.

Try all of the non-medicine treatments you are comfortable with and give them time to work. If you are inclined, Chiropractic, acupuncture, massage, and some herbal techniques work well for most headaches. Remember to consider your diet as a possible source of triggers for headaches and remove foods that may cause headaches before you go for the medical options.

Chronic Pain is pain that you have been suffering with for more than a couple of weeks or months. Try to determine the cause of your pain, and write down what makes the pain better or worse during the day. Look at how much sleep you get, how much and what type of work you do, and how that affects your pain.

Try altering your patterns of exertion to see if anything you do makes a difference in your level of pain. Use braces and TENS stimulation or other pain techniques to see if they help before you go to the specialist.

Chiropractic and massage may help. If they don't, you may need the help of a neurologist to determine the source and possible remedy for your pain. Visit with your primary care doctor to get the referral necessary for most insurance companies, and follow through with the doctor's advice.

Dizziness (vertigo) is a sensation you get where the room may spin around you, or you may feel unsteady as if you feel you are being spun in the room. Either of these problems can be extremely scary, and can be dangerous if the sensation happens when the person is driving or needs to be focused.

Many times this sensation is the result of a disturbance in the inner ear. This may be caused by sinus pressure, or it may be a deeper problem which will require more expert evaluation. Note the time and circumstance of the dizziness, and note anything you do that makes you more or less dizzy. Try to remember when you were first dizzy and how many times you get dizzy per week.

Numbness or tingling are signs of deeper problems and should not be taken lightly in any circumstance. The reason for this is simple. Nerves are not easily repaired. If you damage a nerve, and the nerve is damaged for just a short time, your loss of function could be permanent.

We have many patients tell us, "I thought this would go away." With nerve problems this is a dangerous attitude, especially if you lose bowel or bladder function. The loss of any function is a big deal, but ***bowel and bladder loss is a medical emergency!***

Weakness is another sign that you need expert help immediately. Weakness that is sudden and has no known cause, such as an injury, is a big deal that needs an expert evaluation. Do not assume you will heal in time, and don't avoid the doctor because you don't want or fear bad news! The sooner you get a proper diagnosis, the better your result will be.

Sudden weakness may indicate damage to your nerve system, it may indicate an underlying disease, or it may simply be the result of a vitamin or mineral deficiency. Tell your doctor all of the important information. Track when the problem started, what makes it better or worse, and be sure to tell him all of the drugs you take and how they affect you.

Movement disorders or seizures almost always require an evaluation by a neurologist. Do not let these problems go untreated or go very long without an examination. Seizures can be treated most of the time, and movement disorders may be helped with drugs or new therapies, which will give you your life back!

Vision problems are another problem that you must not ignore. Most people value their vision and this is rarely a problem that will go on for very long without some type of evaluation, but we have seen people who lost their vision gradually over time and did not notice until it was too late to restore their loss.

Gradual vision loss is dangerous because the victim may not be aware of the loss until they are nearly blind. Pressure in the eye may affect the optic nerve, which will result in permanent vision loss in a short period of time. Other types of vision loss may indicate brain disorders or diseases of the eye that require quick and accurate diagnosis and treatment. (http://www.eyeinstitute.co.nz/the-eye/eye-problems-and-symptoms/sudden-blindness.htm)

Alzheimer's Disease is a neurologic disease of "old age" that has some very distinctive problems and signs. Alzheimer's occurs when people age and they begin to have problems with their memory. This disease begins slowly at first and then can progress. The early signs of Alzheimer's may be subtle and can be easily missed by most people.

In our family, we had a person who suffered with Alzheimer's. One of the very first signs in this person was the inability to understand the rules of a simple card game called "Uno." She simply couldn't get how the number and color rules of the game worked, even though the game is designed for children.

After several months, the signs of a disease may become more apparent, and people close to the affected person may notice more loss of memory and ability. As Alzheimer's progresses, victims show more problems with daily life and memory.

This happens as a result of the brain changes that are unique to Alzheimer's. After an examination, which may include an MRI (magnetic resonance imaging), the person will be assessed for loss of memory and function. This loss is due in great part to brain changes which occur as a part of Alzheimer's.

There are several changes that occur in the brain of a person affected with Alzheimer's. All of the changes in the structure of the brain result in a loss of memory, which can also lead to a loss of functional ability. One of the first things that happens in Alzheimer's is a build-up of protein in different parts of the brain. This protein builds up in clumps known as "plaques," which cause a loss of function of the nerves in the brain and may lead to "tangles" of nerve structures. These two problems are the reason for memory loss.

As the plaques and tangles grow in the brain, the normal connections between nerve cells are lost or changed, which causes more memory loss and eventually may cause a loss of function in the organ systems of your body. When these links in the brain are lost, you lose the ability to make new connections and your short-term memory may be affected or even lost. Eventually, these losses affect long-term memory and may result in death in extremely advanced Alzheimer's disease.

The reason the picture is so bleak is simple…Alzheimer's disease causes the nerve cells in the brain (which is the brain itself) to swell, and then the swelling, plaques, and tangles cause the nerves to die. Wherever the cells lose their connections, or die as a result of this process, the memories stored in, and functions controlled by, this area of the brain are lost. The end stage of the disease causes shrinking of the brain, which is the result of nerve cell death and is the final stage of Alzheimer's.

Research has shown the effects of this disease and how it progresses over time. We know how the disease robs a person of their life and their memories, but we do not know how this disease starts or how to stop it. (http://www.alz.org/research/science/alzheimers_research.asp)

The ten signs of early Alzheimer's are:

1. A loss of memory that is unusual for you or the person with Alzheimer's. This means that the affected person can't remember things that were easy to remember before, they lose things easily, or can't remember names of family members, important dates or events.
2. The person may have a harder time doing things that used to be easy. A person who has Alzheimer's may not be able to work in a job they have done for years because they cannot remember the process of completing a task required to do a good job.
3. Trouble starting or finishing daily tasks that were once routine. People affected by Alzheimer's may not be able to drive because they get lost too easily, or they may go to the store and forget to get the only item they went to buy.
4. Confusion with time or place. People with Alzheimer's may forget times and events or may get lost traveling to a previously familiar place.
5. Vision problems. A person with Alzheimer's may have problems with vision that are unusual for their age. This could create problems and could be dangerous in extreme cases…getting lost would be bad, driving while being lost or mistaking the color of a light could cause severe problems.
6. People with Alzheimer's may have problems with speech, and may forget words or phrases and have trouble using new words in conversation or writing. This may cause them to repeat themselves, or they may get stuck in a loop of words or use a phrase endlessly.
7. They may put things away in an unusual place and may accuse those around them of moving a possession or object. This can

also cause them to accuse others of stealing when the object was easily found later. We have reports by family members who were shocked to be accused in this way (sometimes forcefully), and were very hurt when the object was found, but the person with Alzheimer's didn't admit the mistake.

8. Poor judgment and less attention to grooming. There have been many reports of affected people who gave way too much money when asked for a donation or when asked to pay a bill. Grooming becomes a problem for some people who were very tidy before the disease took effect.
9. People with Alzheimer's may withdraw from social interaction and may avoid any new events or contacts with unfamiliar people. In the advanced stages of the disease, the person may not be able to remember children or family members who they have known all their lives. During the late stages of the disease, our family member often did not know who I was, even though she had known me for over five years. I could tell when she was confused; and even at times seemed scared or lost her place just by losing her attention on what she was doing.
10. Changes in mood or behavior. Patients with Alzheimer's become upset easily and may express unusual mood swings rapidly. Our family member had a specific challenge remembering when the dishes in the dishwasher were clean or dirty and got very upset when she was told she was wrong. Using visual aids, such as a magnetic sign that says "Dirty" or "Clean," helps with simple problems like this one. But the reason behind the mood change is the brain changes stop the normal mechanism (in the limbic system) that helps us to keep our anger in check when we feel challenged or attacked. (http://www.alz.org/alzheimers_disease_10_signs_of_alzheimers.asp)

Now that you know all of the early signs of Alzheimer's disease, what do you do with the information? The truth of the matter is, you won't do ***anything*** until you, or someone you know, begins to show the signs of the disease! Then, you'll do exactly what we did, you'll search and dig for every morsel of information you can get to give you some hope of beating this disease.

Unfortunately, this doesn't help very much after the diagnosis has been made! We all need to do what we can ***before Alzheimer's is diagnosed to have any chance at beating the disease!*** We have heard for many years that nothing we do will prevent or slow Alzheimer's, but now new research is showing the opposite. We may not be able to stop the disease, but if we are diligent and follow through with a plan, we can slow and possibly even stop the onset of the disease!

Action Plan to Slow Alzheimer's

1. Current research shows that there are many factors that contribute to Alzheimer's. Your age, the genes you inherit, where you live and work, your lifestyle, and any medical problems you may have may affect how and when Alzheimer's will strike, or if it will strike you at all. ***The only two you can't control are age and genetics. The rest can be influenced to help you lessen your chances for Alzheimer's.***
2. Unfortunately, there are no treatments (drug treatments) that work to stop Alzheimer's, and there are no tests that will give you an accurate warning (yet). However, as medicine advances, we may soon have tests and/or treatments that will be of some use to Alzheimer's victims.
3. Remember the connection between your heart and your brain! When you think of Alzheimer's, think of the things you may do that affect your heart. Because your brain gets nutrition from your blood, anything that hurts your heart will also hurt your brain! Some studies have shown that up to 80% of people diagnosed with Alzheimer's also had heart disease! This may mean that even with the tangles and plaques found in the brain during the disease, the disease may not be as bad (and/or may not develop) if there is no heart disease in the patient.
4. Physical exercise and diet are vitally important to help your circulation and nourish your brain. Diet and exercise decrease heart-related disease and stop plaque from developing in your blood vessels. A Mediterranean diet, which reduces red meat and focuses on whole grains, fruits and vegetables, seafood, olive oil and nuts, is a good way to begin for most people. Exercise to get

your heart beating will also help keep your blood vessels clear.

5. Make sure you do not hit your head or suffer unnecessary head trauma. This may sound like fairly obvious advice, but head trauma can cause damage to the brain which will only make Alzheimer's worse. Anything that would negatively impact your brain should be avoided at all costs. If you love contact sports, or snow skiing or boarding, always wear a helmet!
6. Maintain social interaction and keep learning. Since one of the signs of Alzheimer's is a loss of social contacts and loss of memory, it only makes good sense to keep learning and keep interacting with others. This forces your brain to maintain connections and pathways that may otherwise be destroyed! (http://www.alz.org/research/science/alzheimers_prevention_and_risk.asp)
7. Make sure you monitor your progress with a professional and keep tabs on how your medicines work for you! We found that standard use of the prescribed medicines for our family member did not work as hoped, and her medications had to be adjusted to give her better results.
8. Make sure you have planned for all outcomes! Give specific directions to anyone who is given medical power of attorney for your care if you become unable to make decisions for yourself.
9. Keep up with current treatments! Medicine makes new discoveries every year. A new drug therapy or a new treatment may offer help in the near future, so keep searching online for any help.

New research in Regenerative Medicine has shown some benefit for patients with stem cell therapy. Look locally for qualified professionals who may be able to help with this type of intervention. The quicker you get a correct diagnosis and begin treatment, the better your long-term picture and health will be.

13
High Blood Pressure

High blood pressure (hypertension) is a condition that is dangerous on many different levels. The real problem with high blood pressure is it may not have symptoms that the affected person is aware of during the disease. We used to think high blood pressure would cause symptoms like headaches, dizziness, flushing of the face, or may even cause blood vessels in the eyes to burst.

The truth is, none of these things may happen in a person who has high blood pressure. There are studies that have shown that people with high blood pressure have ***fewer headaches*** than people with normal blood pressure! It is vital for you to know your blood pressure numbers, and the only way to know your numbers is to get checked. (http://www.heart.org/HEARTORG/Conditions/HighBloodPressure/SymptomsDiagnosisMonitoringofHighBloodPressure/What-are-the-Symptoms-of-High-Blood-Pressure_UCM_301871_Article.jsp)

It is vital for you to know your blood pressure numbers, and the only way to know you numbers is to get checked.

Blood pressure readings have two different numbers that represent different events. The first (top) number is called the "systolic pressure" and s***hould be under 120mm Hg*** (that's 120 millimeters of mercury pressure) in "normal" people. It is the amount of pressure inside of the artery measured when the heart is actively pushing blood through the vessels (when the left ventricle is contracting).

The second (bottom) number should be much lower than 120mm Hg, in fact, this number should be under ***80 mm Hg*** to be considered "normal." This number is called the "diastolic pressure" and represents the pressure inside of the arteries of your body when the heart is not beating. These two numbers, when too high, can damage your heart and other organs and cause problems in the smaller vessels which may lead to a dangerous stroke (brain attack).

Recently, these numbers have been increased for people as they age. New guidelines from the American Medical Association were adjusted because there was little evidence that taking blood pressure medicine helped as much as previously thought. Now your blood pressure target should be 140mm Hg on the high side and 90mm Hg on the low side if you are under 60 years old. (http://www.webmd.com/hypertension-high-blood-pressure/news/20140329/new-blood-pressure-guidelines-may-take-millions-of-americans-off-meds)

The new guidelines also allow those with no medical problems over the age of 60 to go up to 150mm Hg on the high side and 90mm Hg on the low side. Don't discontinue any medication you take without the advice and consent of your doctor. If you have any disease that affects your kidneys or other vital organs (your heart, brain, liver or lungs), get advice from your doctor to see what you need to do to maintain your health.

A stroke (now being called a brain attack) is very dangerous and can cause death in a person if not recognized and treated quickly. A stroke happens when a blood vessel ruptures in the brain and then damages brain tissue. The damage results from a loss of oxygen to the part of the brain where the stroke occurs. The biggest problem with a stroke is the person who is affected may not even recognize or understand what has happened. (http://www.medicalnewstoday.com/articles/7624.php)

Strokes usually can be treated if the person makes it to a hospital for care ***quickly!*** You must help the person who is having a stroke because if they do not get care, the damage done by the lack of blood flow and loss of oxygen may be permanent within hours of the stroke. The new acronym we use to recognize and act is called **FAST**.

F - Face: look for drooping on one side of the person's face (ask them to smile and see if both sides of their face curve up).

A - Arms: ask the person to raise both arms up in the air. If one arm drops quickly, or cannot be raised at all, suspect a stroke!

S - Speak: ask the person to talk. If they have problems speaking with either of the two signs above…

T - Time: to call 9-1-1! Do not delay or hesitate, call 9-1-1! Even if you are wrong, you may still save the person's life from another problem. (http://www.strokeassociation.org/STROKEORG/WarningSigns/Stroke-Warning-Signs-and-Symptoms_UCM_308528_SubHomePage.jsp#)

My wife was getting her grandparents ready to go to the doctor when her grandmother suddenly went limp. She called me and said she thought her grandmother was having a stroke. I immediately asked her to do the FAST check, but told her to call 9-1-1 first! Elderly people get ill and may die quickly if not treated quickly. Her grandmother was not having a stroke, but she was having a heart attack! My wife's quick actions saved her grandmother's life!

High blood pressure can cause "end organ damage."

High blood pressure can cause "end organ damage." This means that the organs (such as the heart, liver, and kidneys) may be damaged when the blood pressure gets too high. This damage may occur at any age! When young people get high blood pressure, it is usually caused by other diseases, or by heredity, but high blood pressure in young people is almost always an indicator of future problems like a heart attack. (http://www.mayoclinic.org/diseases-conditions/high-blood-pressure-in-children/basics/causes/con-20033799)

Causes of High Blood Pressure

Primary High Blood Pressure (Essential Hypertension) - This type of blood pressure disease results from many different factors. You may have a build-up of fatty deposits in the arteries, a thickening of the arteries, or narrowing or contracting of the smaller arteries in your body, which drives your blood pressure higher than it should be. This type of hypertension develops over the years and the most dangerous part of this condition is the lack of outward signs that a disease is damaging your body. This is the type of high blood pressure that affects most adults. (http://www.mayoclinic.org/diseases-conditions/high-blood-pressure/basics/causes/con-20019580)

Secondary High Blood Pressure (Secondary Hypertension) - Although the main cause of high blood pressure is still unknown in science, many different factors are known to make it worse, and blood pressure may be controlled if you take control and responsibility for your own health. One of the first things we look at with patients who suffer with high blood pressure is weight. If you weigh too much, your blood pressure may be high as a result of the increased stress on your body and your heart from carrying the extra weight!

Sometimes people get sensitive when they feel they are being confronted about their weight or their appearance. The way I like to handle the weight issue with most of my patients is by letting them know that I struggle with my weight all of the time, too. Then I ask them if they think they could walk up and down the stairs with 20 pounds in each hand. Most of the patients who have a weight problem will confess that they can't. Then I point out to them that this is exactly what they are putting their body and heart through when they carry an extra 40 pounds of weight around.

When you get control of your weight, you get control of your life and you may even find yourself enjoying it a bit more! I'm not saying that you have to be thin to enjoy your life, but there are many things you may not be able to do if your weight is out of control.

Smoking is well known to cause narrowing of the arteries and this may cause your blood pressure to rise, especially if you smoke actively for many years. Most of us know that smoking will damage your lungs, leads to cancer, and causes other diseases and birth defects, but many people are not aware that smoking can cause an increase in your blood pressure.

Smoking may cause heart disease and is documented in many studies to raise blood pressure during the act of smoking, and the effects of the nicotine can last for several minutes. Smoking may also increase the plaque in the arteries of those who smoke for a long time or are continuously exposed to second-hand smoke. (http://www.heart.org/HEARTORG/Conditions/HighBloodPressure/PreventionTreatmentofHighBloodPressure/Tobacco-and-Blood-Pressure_UCM_301886_Article.jsp)

The real way to manage high blood pressure is to focus on your lifestyle and make better choices. But if you do all of the right things and still have high blood pressure, you will need the help of a doctor, and you will need medicine to get your pressure under control. Here is a list of the common medicines for high blood pressure and how they work to lower your pressure.

Drugs to lower high blood pressure

Angiotensin Converting Enzyme (ACE) Inhibitors - This is a medicine that works to lower blood pressure by blocking the production of a chemical in your body (angiotensin II), which causes your blood vessels to contract and drives your blood pressure higher. ACE inhibitors work by blocking the enzyme that causes conversion of angiotensin I, slowing the conversion of angiotensin I to angiotensin II. This opens the blood vessels and lowers your blood pressure.

These drugs are not to be used for people who are pregnant, or who already have narrowing of the renal arteries. They may cause birth defects in pregnant women, and may cause more problems with kidney function in people who already have kidney problems.

Side Effects - most common side effects are cough, high blood potassium levels, low blood pressure, which can lead to dizziness, headache, drowsiness, weakness, rash, flushing of the face, or a salty or metallic taste in the mouth. If you have swelling of the lips or other tissues, nausea, vomiting, or problems breathing, you could be allergic or sensitive to the drug and it should be avoided in the future.

The effects of ACE inhibitors may be decreased by drugs like aspirin, ibuprofen, indomethacin, and naproxen. Because ACE inhibitors may increase your blood level of potassium, you should be careful if you are taking potassium (or salt substitutes which may contain potassium) supplements with ACE inhibitors. These drugs can also increase the level of lithium in your blood if you take lithium for any reason. (http://www.medicinenet.com/ace_inhibitors/page2.htm#what_are_the_side_effects_of_ace_inhibitors)

Angiotensin II Receptor Blockers (ARBs) - These drugs block or inhibit a substance in your body that will cause the blood vessels to constrict, driving your blood pressure higher. Normally, the liver releases a hormone in the body called angiotensinogen, which is changed into angiotensin when the kidney secretes renin (an enzyme) if the blood pressure is too low. These drugs make the blood vessels widen and relax, making it easier for the blood to pass through (less pressure). ARBs also help by getting more salt and water into the urine by working directly on the hormones that regulate salt and water in your body.

ARBs are used in heart failure patients, or in patients who don't like the cough that may occur when they use an ACE inhibitor. ARBs can also slow or stop kidney damage in patients who have kidney disease, or whose kidneys may have signs or symptoms of early damage from or with type 2 diabetes.

Side Effects - ARBs have side effects very similar to the other blood pressure medications. Most commonly, patients may experience coughing (although not as bad as the coughing from ACE inhibitor use), higher blood potassium levels, low blood pressure, drowsiness, dizziness, a salty or metallic taste in the mouth, and sexual dysfunction. ARBs are not recommended for patients who are pregnant, as they may cause birth defects. If you have swelling of the lips or tongue, experience itching, or have any other signs of an allergy to this or any other drug, stop taking the drug and call 9-1-1. (http://www.uptodate.com/contents/actions-of-angiotensin-ii-on-the-heart)

Beta Blockers - Beta blockers work in your body by blocking the effects that the hormone adrenaline has on your heart. Adrenaline is secreted from the inside of the adrenal gland (medulla), which is a gland that sits on top of your kidneys. When you get excited, or need more blood in the muscles of your body, the adrenal glands make and secrete adrenaline (epinephrine), which helps allow more blood flow to the muscles of your body. In your heart, it increases the flow of blood and may lead to higher blood pressure.

Beta blockers work by preventing the effect of adrenaline that lowers your blood pressure. Doctors won't usually prescribe this drug for blood pressure without another drug, because the action of the drug is short-lived in your body (half-life), and this means the drug must be taken repeatedly to make your blood pressure low and prevent heart damage.

Doctors may use this drug for a variety of reasons. Beta blockers may be used for high blood pressure, chest pain, migraine headaches, heart failure, glaucoma (the pressure in the eye is too high, which may cause blindness), anxiety, hyperthyroidism, and other medical problems. Make sure if you take beta blockers that you continue to take other medications you have been prescribed, and always tell your health care provider all of the other medications you take!

Side Effects - Beta blockers may cause fatigue, cold hands and feet, headache (which is weird, because it is used to treat migraines), upset stomach, constipation, diarrhea, dizziness, shortness of breath, trouble sleeping, low sex drive or depression. These drugs do not work as well on some black people (no one knows why), so make sure you are getting the right drug for the right reason!

Calcium Channel Blockers (CCBs) - These drugs are used to lower high blood pressure, and they work by blocking the effect of calcium on the muscle cells in your heart. Calcium makes electrical conduction of signals from cell to cell in the heart muscle cells possible. In your heart, the electrical signals flow like a wave from one cell to another, and give the heart the ability to conduct a wave-like impulse that helps to squeeze the blood from one chamber of your heart to the next. This action allows your heart to efficiently pump the blood from the heart to the lungs, and out to the body for circulation.

Calcium also causes contraction of the cells in the arteries, which widens (dilates) the arteries and makes it easier for the heart to pump blood. When the arteries are open (wider), the heart uses less force to push the blood through the body, and the blood pressure is lowered. If the heart works less to push the blood out, it uses less oxygen and the net effect is better for the heart. When your heart works less, the heart gets more blood to the muscles and cells in the heart, and this is more ideal for a healthy heart!

CCBs are used to treat high blood pressure, abnormal heart rhythms, angina (the cramping chest pain experienced during a cardiac episode), migraine prevention, and other heart/vascular problems like Raynaud's disease and cardiomyopathy (disease of the heart muscle). Verapamil and diltiazem are CCBs that are used mainly to treat heart rhythm problems. Amlodipine is preferred when heart failure (which is when the heart stops working well or is close to stopping) is the problem, and the arteries of the heart need to be dilated or opened to prevent further damage to your heart.

Side Effects - Common side effects of these drugs include headaches, flushing of your skin, swelling of your arms or legs, drowsiness, low blood pressure and dizziness. If you develop a rash, or have swelling of the face, lips or your tongue, you should stop the drug immediately and call 9-1-1! These drugs do interact with other drugs, so you must make sure to tell your doctor, or the person who writes your prescription, about all your other medicines. (http://www.rxlist.com/script/main/art.asp?articlekey=94662)

Diuretics - Diuretics are drugs that cause the water in your body to be removed through your kidneys. The diuretics are drugs that make salt (sodium) move through the kidneys and out into the urine. As the salt goes, it takes water with it. This decrease in water and salt makes your blood pressure lower. Simply put, less water and less salt means less fluid, and less fluid means lower blood pressure!

There are three different types of diuretics: thiazide, loop, and potassium-sparing diuretics. Each one of these drugs works on a different part of your kidneys, and each has different uses as well as different side effects. These drugs are recommended by most doctors as the first drugs used to treat high blood pressure in most patients. Diuretics are generally safe, and have fewer side effects than other medications.

Side Effects - Diuretics have common side effects that include frequent or increased urination, too much potassium in your blood (with a potassium-sparing medicine like aldactone or inspra), too little potassium in your blood (when taking a thiazide such as chlorthiazide, or hydrochlrothiazide), low blood levels of sodium, dizziness, headaches, increased thirst, cramping of your muscles, increased blood sugar or cholesterol, skin rash, joint disorders like gout, impotence or menstrual irregularities. Diuretics have generally fewer side effects and are well tolerated by most people. Make sure you understand how to use this drug and check to see if any other drugs you are taking may interact with this drug. (http://www.mayoclinic.org/diseases-conditions/high-blood-pressure/in-depth/diuretics/art-20048129?pg=1)

Action Plan for High Blood Pressure

1. Know what kind of high blood pressure you have. Check your blood pressure daily, before you have any coffee or tea. We ask our patients to check their blood pressure first thing in the morning to get a baseline.
2. If your blood pressure is high, know your numbers! Remember, 120/80 is your goal unless you have other diseases which complicate your health and make this number unrealistic. Take your medication regularly and at the same time each day. Ask your doctor if you can take your medicine at night if it keeps you from sleeping (waking up to pee can cost you valuable sleep). Remember, the new guidelines as you age mean you may have blood pressure of up to 150/90 if you are older than 60 with no health problems.
3. Get your weight under control by eating right and begin a doctor-approved exercise program. Make sure you include your doctor in any decisions you make to change your health, especially if you decide to discontinue a prescribed medicine for any reason!
4. Understand how your medicines work and make sure you tell your doctor ***all of the medicines you take and what they are for!*** Be aware of any and all drug interactions and side effects.
5. If your blood pressure remains high, even if you are taking your medicines regularly, you must go to the doctor for help! High blood pressure can cause major damage to the organs in your body, and can cause a stroke which could kill you! Don't let any of these problems develop by failing to get needed help.

14

Headaches

Headaches are one of the most common types of pain that most people experience. If you've never had a headache, consider yourself extremely lucky! There are many different types of headaches, but there are three main classes of headaches. To make this as simple as possible, we'll focus on the three main headache classes.

Headaches may be broken down into primary headaches, secondary headaches, and other types of headaches including cranial and facial pain. Obviously, any head pain may be called a headache. But the most common definition of a headache is pain that originates from the upper neck, or the head. When you have a headache, your head may feel like it might explode, but the truth is, the brain itself has no pain fibers, so the pain doesn't generally originate from your brain.

Primary Headaches - Primary headaches can be divided into migraines, cluster headaches, and tension headaches.

The most common type of headache most people experience is the **tension headache**. Tension headaches occur in women more than men, but studies indicate that 1 in 20 people may suffer from headaches on a daily basis, and 50% of adults suffered a headache in the last year. It is almost impossible to calculate the amount of productivity lost from a simple headache if 50% of adults suffer from at least one tension headache per year!

Although the cause of tension headaches is unknown, the main factors that contribute to tension headaches are loss of sleep, poor diet, skipping meals, muscular tension from poor posture, and increased levels of stress. Children may also suffer from stress headaches as a result of changes they experience from school or home environments (http://www.medicinenet.com/tension_headache/article.htm).

Common symptoms of tension headaches are head pain that affectsa a person but does not keep them from normal activity.

Common symptoms of tension headaches are head pain that affects a person but does not keep them from normal activity. Many of our patients tell us that their headache begins as a nagging ache at the back of their head that gets worse as the stress they experience gets worse. This stress can be from any source, but is more commonly from lifestyle activities or work. Some people report they feel like an invisible claw is pulling at the muscles in their neck, and this is the source of their pain.

This type of headache does not usually cause nausea or vomiting in most people. There are some people who report they have light sensitivity and are sensitive to sound when they have a bad tension headache, although this is not common. You can lose sleep from this type of headache, but most tension headaches get

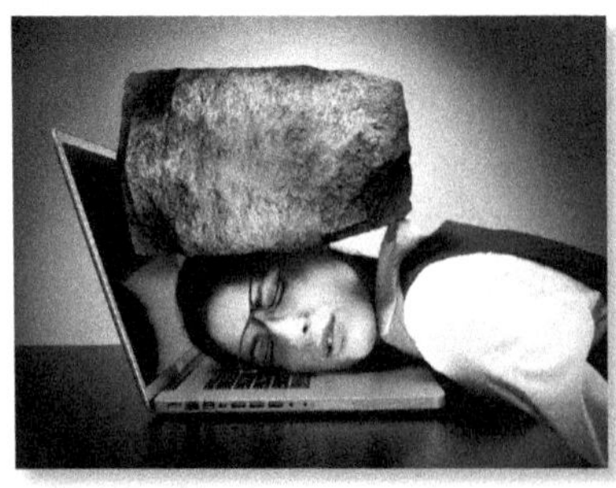

better when you get rest, eat properly, or reduce the amount of stress you have in your life.

Getting a diagnosis from your doctor may be difficult, as there are usually no abnormal findings during the physical exam of someone who suffers with tension headaches. Blood work may be done to make sure you have no other problems that could be causing your headaches, but MRIs or CT scans may be a waste of time and money, as all tests in most people show no problems or causes.

Doctors will often recommend Tylenol, Ibuprofen or aspirin, depending on what a patient can tolerate or what drug works best. Some headaches must be treated with prescription medications to break the cycle of pain. However, we have found much better results and more lasting relief with chiropractic adjustments and muscle work followed by rehabilitation of the spine (we use Active Release Techniques for muscle work). You may also want to try using acupuncture, massage or meditation, or other stress-relief techniques.

The drugs used mostly focus on decreasing swelling and relieving pain. Drugs in this class usually have side effects of bleeding (from the COX interaction), stomach irritation, and rebound headaches if you use the medications too much! Remember not to use these medications if you may be pregnant or if you have any health conditions that put you or your health at risk. (http://www.rxlist.com/tylenol-side-effects-drug-center.htm)

Migraines are well known by most people to be the severe headaches that cause people so much pain they cannot function when the headache strikes. Some people will see auras, smell or hear something before they get a migraine headache. Migraine victims may also be sensitive to some smells or sounds, and may get a migraine if they are exposed to these triggers.

Migraines may also be caused by stress, alcohol or caffeine withdrawal, loss of sleep, changes in hormonal levels in women, exercise, or missed meals. These headaches may also be triggered by common types of foods such as gluten, strawberries, chocolate, coffee, MSG in foods, nitrates in foods or wine, and some fruits like banana, avocado or citrus fruits. It is also worth mentioning that there are a lot of triggers that are unique to the victim. Some people have come to our office and reported sensitivity to things they encountered that are not on any list!

The one thing to keep in mind if you suffer from migraines is to keep track of things that start a headache

The one thing to keep in mind if you suffer from migraines is to keep track of things that start a headache (triggers), and don't wait for the headache to get too bad before you treat the pain. I have had a regular tension headache turn into a migraine because I waited too long to take something for the pain. I don't need to tell you how stupid I feel when this happens, because I should really know better!

Cluster headaches are one-sided headaches that occur in a regular pattern. This type of headache is named a cluster because of the timing of the headaches. People who suffer from this type of headache report they have headaches on a regular frequency. They have chronic repeated headaches that are separated by periods of weeks to months of no headaches. This type of headache is more frequent in men, and may be due to the release of serotonin or histamine in your body. But we still do not know the exact cause of any headache! (http://www.ncbi.nlm.nih.gov/pubmedhealth/PMH0001790/)

Treatments for headaches

I have been in healthcare for a long time. I cannot tell you the number of people we see in our office who have suffered with headaches for years or decades, and have tried literally everything to stop the headaches with no result, who get immediate relief from a simple chiropractic adjustment. This is the first thing I try when I have a headache!

Chiropractic adjustments work by removing nerve irritation and reducing muscle tension that may be the cause of a headache. In our office, whenever someone reports a headache we adjust their neck first (if they can tolerate an adjustment or want one), then try other methods of treatment second! Chiropractic adjustments are effective and ***safe.***

People often treat headaches with simple over-the-counter medications like aspirin, Tylenol, or Ibuprofen. These medications all work by blocking inflammation or swelling, which causes the pounding sensation you get when you have a headache. My favorite is aspirin, because this drug is a pain killer and reduces swelling and is very affordable for most people.

Whatever medication you choose, remember that there are usually less expensive medicines that are available right in your local grocery store. Look at the label and read what the drug is made of! The cheaper drugs may have a bit less of the active ingredient per pill, but they still contain the same medicine!

If your headache is the result of a histamine reaction, this means that you are probably having some type of allergy. Watering eyes and the runny nose may indicate that you need to find out what you are allergic to in order to stop the headache.

Good advice for these headaches is to try an inexpensive anti-histamine that works for you, and see if it helps your headache. If it does, then you know what to do when the headache starts. Don't let these types of headaches get away from you, because the pressure from a histamine headache will build up over time! The allergic substance (pollen, pet dander, or whatever) probably won't go away on its own, so don't waste time waiting for things to get better.

If your headaches don't go away or get better with chiropractic adjustments, over-the-counter medicine, massage, or acupuncture, it's time to go to the doctor to see if you have a deeper cause of your headache. The doctor will do a complete exam, so make sure you tell him everything you have tried to relieve your pain. He may decide to do more tests, or he may give you stronger medication.

Drugs that are commonly prescribed for headaches are used to relieve the pain of a headache or prevent the headache from beginning. Obviously, you should try to treat a headache yourself, unless you have pain that rates as a nine or ten on a scale of one to ten with ten being severe pain.

You already know about NSAIDs, and the drugs you will most likely be prescribed are a combination drug called butalbital/acetaminophen/with or without codeine or caffeine (Fioricet). This combination of drugs helps most migraine victims, but it may also cause side effects like nausea, vomiting, lightheadedness, dizziness, and sensitivity to light (skin). (http://www.drugs.com/sfx/fioricet-side-effects.html)

Other drugs that work for headaches and migraines are topiramate, sumatriptan, amitriptyline, atenolol, ergotamine, metoprolol, propranolol and many others. You should look these drugs up, and be ready to ask your doctor for direction on which drug may work best for you.

Ergotamine (Cafergot) is a strong drug that makes the blood vessels smaller. This may help some people by reducing the nausea which may occur when using other migraine medicines. Many people use ergotamines in combination with other drugs to help reduce nausea, but ergotamine is not as specific for migraines as triptans.

Triptans are drugs that may prevent headaches from coming back. They work by targeting the receptors in your body that make chemicals and lead to migraine headaches. According to research, triptans are just as effective as ergotamines, and may be more migraine-specific.

Midrin is a combination drug containing three different compounds that make the blood vessels smaller, decrease pain, and calm your body's responses. This drug, specifically the drug that makes the blood vessels smaller in the combination, is still under review by the FDA.

Antihistamines may also work to lessen the pain when you have a migraine. When you get a migraine, your body secretes histamines, which dilate the blood vessels. Antihistamines decrease the size of the inflamed blood vessels and may help reduce the pain of your migraine. Your doctor can help you pick the right type of antihistamine for your migraines.

There are no drugs that prevent migraines, but there are certain drugs and herbal compounds that many people use for this purpose. Blood pressure medicines, such as **beta-blockers** and **calcium channel blockers**, lower blood pressure and may help prevent migraines.

Other methods of treating migraines and headaches involve the use of tricyclic antidepressants (Elavil), other depressants like Zoloft or Paxil, anti-seizure medicines (Topamax, Neurontin, or Depakote), and the use of herbal compounds like feverfew and butterbur. If none of these methods work for you, you may want to consider the more aggressive therapies now available that involve injections of Botox, or other therapies such as trigger point injections or electrical implants, if your pain is disabling. (http://www.rxlist.com/migraine_medications/drugs-condition.htm)

After years of migraines, I thought I had done all I could to help myself. I had tried all of the over-the-counter medicines and every remedy I could to prevent my headaches. Then I had a spell of headaches that wouldn't respond to anything! I even got injections of anesthetics (not Botox), but nothing seemed to help.

I felt that I must be missing something, and maybe my headaches were caused by something I was doing (a trigger) that I was missing. I read some research on gluten sensitivity, which listed migraines as a result of gluten sensitivity. So I decided to try getting rid of gluten in my diet for two weeks.

The results were immediate and astounding to me! After this short trial, I had a couple of days where I did not sleep well. This almost always caused a headache and sometimes led to a migraine. But not this time. I had finally found my trigger!

Eliminating gluten has now become my number one go-to when I counsel patients. If they have difficult headaches, they say they have tried everything, and nothing seems to fix the problem…gluten elimination may help. I ask them to try it for two weeks, and many report it works better than any drug!

Whatever treatment you decide, make sure you do the research before you begin treatment to insure you get the results you desire. Many of the treatments require more than one application or dose, and some of these treatments have side effects that you may not like!

There are also treatments that focus on treating your headache or migraine when you are suffering from the headache. Acupuncture or massage may help lessen the effect and pain of a headache, but these options may not get rid of the pain and do not treat the cause. Treatments that do work to stop the pain of a migraine are trigger point injections and nerve blocks.

Trigger point injections and nerve blocks must be done by a qualified doctor or nurse practitioner. The doctor will tell you which drugs he is using in the injection to stop your pain. Some doctors will add steroids to the shots...make sure you tell him/her if you have allergies to any drugs and also tell him if you are diabetic! Steroids will cause problems with sugar levels in diabetic patients and can cause real problems you don't want!

Newer forms of treatment are nerve blocks of the sphenopalatine nerve, and electrode implants which are surgically implanted and deliver an electric pulse to decrease the pain of a migraine. (http://www.dailymail.co.uk/health/article-203244/Implant-switch-migraine.html)

These forms of treatments should be considered a "last resort" for your headaches. Almost everyone who suffers with migraines or headaches will find some relief in the treatments already discussed, but if you still suffer and you have tried everything, look into the newer treatments!

Action Plan for Headaches

1. First you must determine the type of headache you have. Once you have decided the type, look at the treatments you may use and get busy! The first step in treating headaches is always to see if there is an underlying allergy or food sensitivity. If there is, eliminate the food or substance and see if your headaches stop. Then, move on to the next treatment or try a combination of natural therapies before moving on to drug treatments. Remember that gluten is common in a lot of foods and elimination of gluten has helped many people with headaches.
2. The second step is to reduce your stress levels and try massage or chiropractic. I would try all of the easy things before you start any drug therapy. Acupuncture is next if you don't like the massage or chiropractic option. Remember to look at small things like drinking (coffee or alcohol), your posture, and sleeping and work positions! These may add to the mechanical stress and cause headaches.
3. Drug therapy should always begin with over-the-counter drugs! See if plain aspirin will help with your headaches (make sure you are not allergic and do not have ulcers), or try white willow bark if you prefer the more natural option. Move on to the over-the-counter antihistamines, and remember to avoid any drugs that do not work with medicine you already take.
4. Step four is to go to the doctor for help with other drugs. Tell your doctor all of your symptoms! Include what you have already tried (written form is better) and the results. Make sure you understand the medicines he prescribes and the side effects you may experience.

5. Now you need to consider the most aggressive therapies to treat your headaches. Trigger point injections, Botox injections, electrode implants (if your headaches are disabling), or a mix of therapies to get rid of your headaches. I hope you never need this step, but many people find help in this last step

15

Diabetes

Diabetes is a blood sugar disorder that is generally broken down into two types of diabetes. Both types of diabetes have problems with the hormone insulin, which is produced in your pancreas and helps to keep blood sugar levels stable. Type I diabetes is caused when the body does not produce enough insulin in the pancreas. Type II diabetes may develop over the years and may be due to decreasing production of insulin or to insulin resistance.

The reason this is vital to your health is very simple. When you eat any food, the body digests the food and breaks it down into a basic sugar called glucose. This sugar is used for energy in almost every cell in your body. Your body needs a stable supply of glucose to keep you alive and well. Too much sugar in your blood can cause problems in the small blood vessels and this leads to disease. Too little sugar in the blood makes you feel awful (hypoglycemia).

Type 1 Diabetes

Type 1 diabetes is usually diagnosed in children and young adults and has been called juvenile diabetes for as long as I can remember.

It may be managed well and those who are afflicted can live long and productive lives. Type 1 diabetes may have genetic factors that cause the disease, and some research suggests it may be triggered by exposure to certain viruses. (http://www.mayoclinic.org/diseases-conditions/type-1-diabetes/basics/definition/con-200195730)

Type 1 diabetics need to supplement insulin on a daily basis because they do not produce insulin in their pancreas. For some unknown reason, the immune system in a type1 diabetic attacks the beta cells in the pancreas and destroys them. This is why type 1 is an autoimmune disease. (http://diabetes.niddk.nih.gov/dm/pubs/causes/Causes_of_Diabetes_508.pdf)

Some research has shown that type 1 diabetes ***may be*** caused by viruses, but this is not the only cause. However, it develops, this form of diabetes permanently stops the production of insulin in the pancreas and the resulting buildup of sugar in the bloodstream can damage blood vessels and nerve tissue, which can cause organ damage or lead to the amputation of limbs damaged by the effects of high sugar.

There is a new procedure for type 1 diabetes called pancreatic transplantation. The surgery replaces a non-functional pancreas with one from an organ donor (who has died). Your old pancreas still produces digestive enzymes necessary for health, but the donor pancreas will produce insulin and may allow you to stop or reduce the use of insulin and other medical therapies to deal with your diabetes.

There are risks and side effects associated with all types of organ replacement. Most notably, transplant patients need to take anti-rejection drugs. These powerful drugs almost always cause a suppression of the immune system, which may cause the patient to become ill from bacterial or viral infections and may increase the risk of cancer.

Studies have been conducted that reveal some transplant patients require fewer anti-rejection drugs, and others may be "weaned" off the drugs and experience little problems with their "new organs." This suggests that all patients may one day be able to tolerate organ transplant or replacement with the same result! (http://www.upmc.com/services/transplant/abdominal-transplants/starzl-institute/pages/drug-weaning.aspx)

The other thing you need to know regarding transplant therapy is these procedures are usually done when every other option has failed. You will probably already have kidney damage if this is a last ditch effort to cure your diabetes. The lesson here is to get help early and avoid the costs and suffering you must endure with a transplant.

If you or someone you love has type 1 diabetes, make sure to educate yourself on the disease and take care of yourself! The biggest stress we see in those who have family members with a disease is they forget that they cannot help someone unless they are healthy. That being said, there is a lot of information on the web about how to set things up so the caregiver doesn't suffer while taking care of another person with a disease. It is possible to have a long, healthy life while managing diabetes! (http://www.diabetes.org/)

Type 2 Diabetes

My father developed type 2 diabetes as he aged. He was a very healthy young man and could hold his own with anyone his age. He flew airplanes (and still does), but he had one small vice. He kept a bag of Hershey's chocolate in his bedside table and ate some candy almost every day.

As he aged, he began to notice little things. He became a little overweight, developed high blood pressure, complained of being tired, and began to notice more frequent trips to the bathroom and dark spots on his skin. These were all signs he was trending towards type 2 diabetes.

What happened to my father can easily happen to anyone. As we age, our body does not do the things we think it should. I noticed that I was no longer able to lose weight as easily after I turned 42 years of age. Many of our patients report the same problems. We simply must pay closer attention to things we were able to do as children with little or no consequences!

Diabetes is a very serious condition. There are three main problems that we see in patients that signal they may be developing diabetes. First, patients report they don't feel well, and they are constantly thirsty, even after they have a drink of water (polydypsia). Then they notice they are hungry and they can't lose weight easily, even if they cut calories (polyphagia). Third, they report that they need to go to the bathroom more often to pee (polyuria). These three problems are called the three "P's" of diabetes.

This is the reason that diabetes and weight are so tightly linked! It is also why diabetes is a very serious problem in health care.

There are some things that we know about diabetes, and a lot we don't know in medicine regarding this disease. First, there are a few signs that you may be at risk for developing diabetes.

Weight - if your weight is hard to control, or you begin to experience hunger that is not satisfied from your normal diet, consider yourself at risk.

Fat distribution - as bad as this seems, if your body fat accumulates around your waist and hips (like mine does), then you are at increased risk for diabetes.

Family history - if anyone in your immediate family (mom, dad, brothers or sisters) has diabetes, your risk goes up!

Race - for some reason we don't understand, ethnicity makes a difference in diabetes. Black, Hispanic, American-Indian and Asian-Americans are more prone to diabetes than are whites.

Age - the older you are, the more you are at risk for diabetes. It could be that most people exercise less as they get older, or that your body loses some of its muscle mass as you age, but older people (over 45) have a higher risk for diabetes.

Metabolic resistance - in this condition, your body develops a resistance to the insulin produced by your pancreas. This results in weight gain (even if you change the way you eat), and higher blood sugar, which leads to diabetes. (http://www.mayoclinic.org/diseases-conditions/type-2-diabetes/basics/risk-factors/con-20031902)

There are other risk factors, but these are the major factors that may indicate you are at risk.

Altering your lifestyle has been proven by research to be the biggest way you can slow down or reverse diabetes.

So, the big question is… "What can I do to prevent type 2 diabetes?" The answer has already been given earlier in the book. But, just for you, I'll repeat it here. Altering your lifestyle has been proven by research to be the biggest way you can slow down or reverse diabetes. Diet and exercise have the most profound effect on blood sugar and, if maintained, can prevent the need for drug therapy. (http://www.ncbi.nlm.nih.gov/pmc/articles/PMC1370926/)

In fact, there are many (some experts) who claim that altering your diet can stop and even end diabetes. Please understand that even though these people have great credentials, you get what you pay for when taking medical advice (even from me) without the benefit of a proper exam. In some cases, free advice may give little to no results!

Patients often tell me that they are confused from the information in books and on the Internet. For those of you (like me) who want a simple way to look at diet, let me distill the information down to an easy to remember formula. If it's white, it ain't right! Anything that is white (flour, rice, potatoes, crackers, pasta, chips, and SUGAR) should be left out of a normal, healthy diet. Anything that converts to sugar quickly in the body also should be avoided.

This means you should eat fresh food! Vegetables, meats, fruit and nuts (as long as you have no allergies) should be eaten daily and regularly to prevent hunger and feed your body. Add exercise to the mix, and you will maintain a proper weight with little to no effort on your part! We have actually had patients who were on insulin and were able to reduce the dose or (in rare cases) get off most of their medications after they controlled their weight!

Under the care of most doctors, you may find that if you begin your care and do as directed by your medical doctor, you will be on drugs for a very long time! Most likely, for the rest of your life.

You may wish to try some of the advice on the Internet, but if your diabetes still causes problems, you will need to consult a doctor. The first thing the doctor will do is get a thorough history from you, including your family history (a family history of diabetes is important). Then he will do a complete examination to make sure you have no other more pressing issues. (http://www.joybauer.com/type-2-diabetes.aspx)

After your examination he will order tests to see if your blood sugar is a problem. The main test for diabetes is A1C. This test is very accurate and will tell the doctor how you have been handling your blood sugar for the last 90 days. This is important, because if you have been having problems it affects the organs of your body and causes disease as you age.

Other tests that are vital involve the other organs of your body. You may find that your diabetes is also part of a complex picture that can also include thyroid issues, high blood pressure, kidney or liver disease, and heart problems. These may be woven together in a disease complex, or the diseases may work against you to prevent you from being healthy and happy.

Whatever the results, please make sure that you get as much information about your condition as you can and begin the process of getting better day by day! There are people who have wonderful stories of healing from almost any disease. Find these sources of inspiration and do not let any disease be a death sentence!

Action Plan for Diabetes

1. Recognize the early signs of diabetes. Type I (juvenile) diabetes usually affects younger people and causes weight loss. Type II diabetes is called "adult onset diabetes" and may cause weight gain.
2. Understand that diabetes may affect your entire body and develop an action plan for dealing with the disease. The first step should be to get your blood work done and make sure that your doctor checks your thyroid! Make sure you understand how your thyroid may drive diabetes, and if this is an issue for you, correct the thyroid first.
3. Learn everything you can about nutrition. The main way to curb diabetes in most people is with proper nutrition. Eliminate empty calories from sugar and foods that convert quickly to sugar (rice, potatoes, bread and pasta). Try eliminating gluten from your diet to help your thyroid and remove toxins from your body.
4. If your diabetes does not respond to these steps, go to the doctor! You will need the advice of an endocrinologist. He/she may be able to help you treat your diabetes without drugs…if you get into the office early enough!
5. Remember that diabetes can be deadly. ***Never*** try to treat yourself by using medication that your doctor did not prescribe and never stop taking medication without telling your doctor. Many people have died trying to self-regulate a medication (taking medicine only when they feel bad, even when the doctor tells them they need the medicine).

15

Do the Right Thing

Every day millions of people go to the doctor for different reasons. Some people are sick and hope the doctor will cure them of illness or disease. Others are trying to manage their health or prolong their life.

Whatever your reason, you need to make the decision that you will either do what your doctor asks you to do, or you won't. As a health care provider, I am constantly shocked when I give solid advice only to find out later that my advice was ignored by the patient.

I was in my office one day and was surprised to see a woman in the front filling out paperwork. She was upset and was crying as she struggled to write. I walked out and asked her if there was anything I could do to help. She looked at me and said, "No, thank you. I'm just upset being here… Do you remember John X? He was my husband."

I replied, "Yes, I remember him. Is he why you're upset?"

She continued, "Yes, he was a patient here. You told him he had high blood pressure and you warned him that if he didn't take his medicine, he might die from a stroke or heart attack…he died last month. You were the only one who told him how bad things could get."

I was shocked to find out one of my patients had died from not taking a simple pill to lower his blood pressure. I hate giving people bad news and I really hate telling people that they must take medication. But, when I give this type of advice, there is usually no other option.

I have told you to get a second and even a third opinion if you need surgery. But, if you are sick or ill and you know something is wrong and your body cannot correct the problem, the only option for you is medicine!

We now live longer and, hopefully, better lives thanks to advances in medical treatments. Some of these treatments are not all they are supposed to be. You can go online right now and see stories of people who are addicted to drugs and surgery. Some of these people have lost their lives in pursuit of the idea that if some drugs or surgery is good, then more drugs and surgery must be better. This addictive personality trait is bad news for anyone!

But, if one doctor tells you that you have a treatable disease that can be managed or eliminated if you do a simple thing like diet or take a pill…PLEASE take the advice. Don't end your life and leave those who love you to suffer from your loss. Get a second opinion if you like, but don't spend your money and waste your time going to the doctor and then ignore his/her advice!

I have known medical doctors and nurses who think they know better because they work in medicine. These people hand out sage advice all day and may even save lives doing their work. But, when given advice that they must take medicine or have surgery, suddenly the rules don't apply. I know a doctor who had his hip replaced and developed an infection (MRSE) after his surgery. Even though the infection could end his life, he refused to take his medicine.

This is an example of how far we will go to justify our own actions. Doctors are the worst patients. I have had many doctors who have come to me for my "special abilities." I am always surprised how difficult it is to get them to do simple things necessary to make themselves better.

You are definitely the only one in control of you. With that knowledge you now have a choice. Act on the advice you paid good money to get, or suffer the consequences of your inaction.

Good advice is not brain surgery, unless the advice is to have brain surgery!

You now know everything you need to know about how to help yourself get the medical care you deserve without spending your last dime getting it. I have written down action plans for you in the areas that trouble people the most over the span of a lifetime. If you have made it this far, you now have a choice…act on the information, or keep doing what you've been doing.

In our office, I look at every person as a family member. When I give them a report of findings, I tell them they have two choices for care. They can "patch the problem or fix the problem." There is only one choice for the person who wants a magical life! Patching a leaking tire on a car may only get you to the next rest stop. Fixing the tire may cost more and may take more time, but you can go much farther after the fix!

Your Final Action Plan

1. If you have a problem, especially a medical problem, recognize that sometimes the only solution may be medicine or surgery.
2. Do your homework and make sure you design the outcome you want before you begin. If your goal is attainable, work until you have met your goal or change the goal for a good reason.
3. Understand the limits of your body are subject to time. As we age, we suffer because of the things we have done in the past. Do your best to get the best result and don't dwell on the past. Things may change for the better in the future!
4. If you get stuck, get outside of yourself by acting as if you were already the person you hope to be. Make sure you follow the quickest path to your goals, and don't get distracted when things appear difficult. Remember that someone somewhere has a much harder path than you could imagine. There are people in this world with very little hope, and some with no opportunity, who live happy lives in spite of it!
5. Take good advice as if it were your own advice to another person and keep moving forward. No one gets anywhere by looking backwards! Sometimes, we all have to swallow a bitter pill to get better.
6. Remember that no one who is here will get out alive. We will all die of something. The best advice I can give you is to live with passion and love as much of your life as you can!

Your Guide to a Great Visit

1. Paperwork - When you go to the doctor, the people there know you are not there because you couldn't think of a better way to spend your day! If and when you get sick, try not to inflict your bad feelings on those who are there to care for you. We HATE paperwork just as much or more than you do. I have spent literally hundreds of hours trying to decrease the number of forms people have to sign and fill out to get seen. They are REQUIRED to make sure you get checked for everything that is important.
2. To decrease your paperwork, keep a written list of all of your medicines (doses, what you take them for, and the times per day and how long you have been taking them) on a separate piece of paper. Give this to the front desk person for them to copy, or make a copy to give them for your file. Do the same for any surgeries or illnesses you have had over your lifetime!
3. Then, when you get to the section which asks for drugs you take and surgeries or illnesses you have/had, simply write "SEE ATTACHMENT" and you're done! MAKE SURE THAT YOUR LIST IS COMPLETE AND THE DATES ARE INCLUDED FOR ALL DRUGS AND SURGERIES. CARRY A COPY OF THIS IN CASE OF EMERGENCY.
4. Don't edit your responses or assume that your care provider doesn't need to know something they ask about you! Even your massage therapist needs to know if you have implants or surgical devices implanted so they don't hurt you during a massage. Answer every question posed about your health completely AND HONESTLY! I know you might be addicted to something, but if you don't tell me you are, I cannot HELP you!
5. Focus your visit on what you want! Make sure you give the doctor

everything he/she needs to help you, but your visit is for you! Tell him your number one problem and how it affects your life. Let him know what you want to be able to do. Add in the things you have tried, how long you tried them, and how it worked or didn't work for your problem.

6. Follow the advice of the doctor when he gives you care recommendations. If you don't like the treatment, ask if there are any alternatives to the care he recommends. If you don't like the final answer, tell him you won't do what he recommends! Then at least you will get something from the visit. You may decide to switch doctors if his response is unkind or too assertive when he is challenged.
7. Follow through with your care! Don't assume you can just call in for a new prescription or drug for treatment. People are often rude when it comes to medicine. If I treat you for high blood pressure, I NEED TO CHECK to make sure the treatment works! Your word is not enough!

ACTION PLAN REFERENCE

Action Plan - Getting Started

1. Make a list of all of your symptoms and decide how you want the doctor to help you.
2. Make sure you are clear on the following:
   a. how the problem started
   b. what makes you feel better or worse
   c. if there is a specific time of day or night you feel better or worse
   d. what you have done and whether it worked (medicines you took are a must)
   e. how bad is your problem or pain (scale of 1-10, 10 is worst)
   f. be clear on what you want the doctor to address during the visit
3. Make a list of your other health issues and how you are being treated for those issues, and if the treatment is working well.
4. Make a list of your medicines, list your doses, how many times per day you take the drug, and how long you have been using the drug. Include why you are taking the medicine, if it is working, and if you have any of the side effects from taking the drug.
5. **Get a second (or third) opinion for any surgical recommendation. Use only excellent doctors with great references.**

Action Plan for Improved Health

1. Write down your health goals for as long as you think you can commit to the plan. If you can only realistically keep these promises for a day, start with just one day and build on that plan!
2. Look at your bad habits and do the research for what this habit will do to your health if you continue it for the rest of your life. Then see if you can commit to change that one thing for a period of time.
3. Commit to a change as a part of your ***lifestyle***. Don't exchange habits or replace a lifestyle change with something that has no reward, or worse, feels like you are being penalized!
4. Make sure others in your life understand and support your new goals. If you need one, get a buddy who will cheer you on if needed, and who will hold you accountable if you slip up.
5. If you fall back into a bad habit (we all DO), make sure you realize that a slip is only one moment of weakness and not a massive life failure. Start over and begin again with day one, then recommit to success!

Action Plan to Stop Smoking

1. When you make the decision to stop smoking it is a cause for celebration, but don't celebrate in a way that may cause you to smoke! Remember that you have triggers that may cause you to crave a cigarette. Drinking and being around others who smoke will make it harder for you.
2. Dopamine is the hormone you secrete when you smoke a cigarette. This substance is the core of your addiction (as well as nicotine). To get past your addiction, you must stay focused and stay in charge! Write down your commitment to quit, and ask a coach or a buddy to help you in times when you feel the urge to smoke again. (http://bigthink.com/going-mental/your-brain-on-drugs-dopamine-and-addiction)
3. If you can't quit cold-turkey, reduce the number of cigarettes you smoke each day, use NRT or medications to help curb your urges until you can comfortably stop smoking. Try putting your cigarettes in a place that is out of your way so you don't have easy access to a smoke when you get cravings.
4. If you respond better to positive feedback, reward yourself for progress. If negative feedback helps, write a list of all the costs and problems associated with smoking and emphasize the lifetime cost of the cigarettes. Then add in the potential diseases you may develop and look up the cost of these diseases. Remember, you may have more than one disease from smoking, and you may have more costs if you look at the physical damage smoking does to your body and possessions!
5. Track your progress daily and keep after your goal of being smoke-free! Even if it takes you ten years to stop smoking, your body will heal. Never, ever, ever give up! (http://www.becomeanex.org/create-profile.php#

Action Plan for Weight Loss

1. Don't eat sugar, or anything that converts to sugar quickly in your mouth. This includes bread and empty calorie starches (rice, pasta, white potatoes, chips and crackers).
2. Don't starve yourself. When most people diet, they try and fail because they eat too little food. Eat six small meals per day (including regular snacks of nuts and non-tropical fruit). You should eat twice as many vegetable servings as protein, and your protein portions should be smaller than the palm of your hand.
3. Drink water, water, water! No sugar drinks or sodas. We recommend no diet sodas either, but if you must drink soda, drink no-sugar soda. If you use sugar substitutes, we recommend Stevia.
4. Commit to your new lifestyle and recognize that small changes will result in big changes in the future. You can change your body just by changing your mind and by being consistent.
5. Exercise is important, but only do exercise that you will repeat! You only need about 30 minutes per day and it will change you forever! Find something you like (walking, swimming, etc.), then add or change the exercise so your body doesn't stagnate. Use the Internet for help! (http://www.webmd.com/fitness-exercise/ss/slideshow-7-most-effective-exercises)

Action Plan for Colds and Flu

1. Make sure to do all of the things that prevent colds and flu before you get sick. If you are high risk, get vaccinated ***before cold and flu season!***
2. Keep your immune system functioning at its best by exercising and eating right all year long.
3. Use common sense to keep yourself and those who are around you healthy. Wash your hands regularly, eat quality, low-sugar foods, don't share drinks or eat after others, and make sure you keep up your exercise routine!
4. If you get sick, understand your body needs more rest! Sleep is one of the best things you can do to help yourself heal faster! Get plenty of rest and don't rush back to work unless it's absolutely necessary.
5. Make sure to disinfect your toothbrush and go ahead and buy a new one you can use after you are well. Don't sweat the $2.00 for a new toothbrush; it's way better than getting sick again after a cold or flu bout!

Action Plan for Breathing Easy

1. Make sure you understand what ***causes*** your symptoms. Once you understand the cause, you will make much better choices about treatment and prevention measures!
2. Consult with your doctor and have a clear result in mind. Think, "I want to be able to play golf without gasping for breath." Having a result in mind before your visit will give you both a common goal. If he/she doesn't think your goal is attainable, find out why and get a second or third opinion. If everyone is in agreement, you'll need to adjust your goal.
3. Make sure you understand what your medicines do! Don't take anyone's advice except your doctor's, and make sure he/she knows everything you take and when you take it! Then, ***do your own research and confirm how the medicine works on you!*** Remember, we are all different; some people react to medicines or combinations of medicines in different ways. Just because a side effect is listed as uncommon doesn't mean you won't get it!
4. Make sure you take all of your health factors into account! Older people and young people need different doses of medicine, and after a while you may develop a resistance or tolerance to a drug that used to work!
5. If your condition gets worse, ***know when to get help!*** Remember the ABCs of health! Airway, Breathing and Circulation. Your airway and your breathing are vital, and are the first systems to be treated in an emergency for a reason!

Action Plan for Back Problems

1. If you have a back problem, the number one thing you must do is **rest**. I have personally injured myself worse after hurting my back because I could not rest.
2. There are many risks when you try to treat your own back pain. If you have a disc injury, you could make things much worse and suffer more. Ice is always a good place to start, but if ice makes your pain worse, stop using it quickly. Bracing your back to add support is a great idea. I wear a brace in my office to prevent injuries.
   a. Get to the doctor ASAP and get a diagnosis for your pain. If you can, use NSAIDs or aspirin to help decrease your pain. Hot or cold patches may dull your pain, but do not take someone else's medication for pain. I have treated patients who thought a loved one's medication would work, but suffered serious side effects from the drug!
3. I recommend trying chiropractic first, physical therapy or medicine second, and surgery is always the last option for back problems. Remember, you can never get uncut from surgery.
4. If chiropractic, physical therapy and medication don't work (or only work for a short time), you need to get an MRI of the injured part of your back to make sure you do not have an injured disc. If you do, you need the help of an expert surgeon.
5. If you have back surgery, you will need to rehabilitate your back. Make sure your weight stays in an ideal range and continue to help yourself with regular exercise to prevent a new injury from occurring.

Action Plan for Thyroid Problems

1. Look at your symptoms and decide if you think you may have a thyroid problem. Look for the following things to confirm the problem. Do you have: low body temperature; weight gain or loss that does not get better even with a strict diet; low energy even with the proper amount of sleep; hair that is falling out for no reason; low or no sex drive; puffiness in the face, tummy and hips; changes in your skin or a noticeable bump or lump in the lower part of your throat? If you do, you will need to check! Remember, the only way to confirm a thyroid problem is a blood test and eventually a scan (MRI or thyroid ultrasound).
2. Make sure you are taking in the right kinds of supplements. You will need to supplement your diet with iodine (salt with iodine doesn't work). We recommend a product called Iodoral, which has a very good source of iodine and is tolerated very well by most people. (http://store.wellbeinggps.com/product/Iodoral-180-Tabs/Default.aspx?gfid=p32&source=googleshopping&adnet-work=g&adtag1=pla&adtag2=&adcreative=17087792217&ad-position=1o2&admatchtype=&adkeyword=)
3. Try to adjust your diet and make sure you are getting ***quality nutritious food*** over quantity. Avoid gluten, empty carbs (like bread, pasta and rice) and sugar as much as possible to see if your body will correct on its own. If this does not work, it's time to get help from your doctor.
4. Be prepared with all of your information. Tell your doctor what you have done to correct your problem and how long you have been working to correct the problem. Be very specific about as much of the information as you can. Let him know if you have a family history of thyroid problems and if you were sick before your problem started.

5. Get the blood tests that your doctor recommends. Make sure to ask him/her to include: TSH, T3 and T4 (regular and free), reverse T3, Thyroid peroxidase antibodies (TPOAb), and Thyroglobulin antibodies (TGAb). You may also want other tests recommended by other medical experts to get a complete picture of the function of your thyroid. Please do what your doctor recommends! Your thyroid is vital to your health and well-being! (http://www.drbrownstein.com/)

Action Plan for Muscle Injuries

1. Make sure you know why your back or muscles hurt. If you injured yourself during exercise or activity, remember RICE (Rest, Ice, Compression, and Elevation) for the first three days after an injury. Use the best braces or supports to prevent further injury to your back or joints.
2. Know your options for care when you get injured. Get advice from a qualified medical or chiropractic professional and follow the advice!
3. Take advantage of the newer technologies to make sure you get the correct diagnosis (MRI and CT scans). Do everything you can to avoid an unnecessary surgery (of any type).
4. Try Active Release Technique, massage and exercise, to rehabilitate the injury (if possible). A lot of injuries that required surgery in the past do not get surgery today! Explore your options, and make sure to follow through with the care and the advice of your chosen experts. Use the Internet for research and make sure to select care that will meet your goals.
5. Don't begin with exercise unless you are sure or are told exercise will help your injury! Get more than one opinion for any injury that requires surgery, and make sure you research every kind of care before paying for help! This will save you thousands of dollars, and prevent needless suffering caused by the wrong treatment.

Action Plan for Arthritis

1. Know what type of arthritis you are dealing with, and make sure you have all of the information you need regarding your disease. When you seek help from your doctor, understand all of the treatment options and the risks with each type of treatment.
2. Understand the cause of arthritis cannot be cured. This means that you must do everything you can do to lessen the effects of arthritis in your body. Make sure you keep track of how different things affect you. Many patients tell me that they feel worse when a storm is coming (they also say that their doctor doesn't believe them). Keep a written log of what causes your pain to get worse, and make special notes of things that make you feel better!
3. Get rid of sugar, wheat, and milk in your diet. All of these foods can cause swelling and make your arthritis symptoms worse. However, if you do not find that getting rid of a food helps, don't eliminate it if you love it!
4. Exercise as much as you can without hurting yourself. As I age, I use less weight and do more repetition when I work out. Some people will find that just moving is an extreme workout. Don't let anyone push you beyond your limit, and be honest with yourself. You need as much exercise as your body will tolerate!
5. Make a list of all of the drugs you take (even the over-the-counter ones), and check the side effects of all the drugs, making sure to list the combined effects of the drugs. Remember that what you eat is also a factor in how well some drugs work. Don't take any new medicine without understanding how and why you are taking it. If it doesn't work for you, tell your doctor before you stop the medication. (http://www.drugs.com/drug_interactions.html)

Action plan for Acne

1. Make sure you understand what you can do and must do to prevent your skin from breaking out. Adjust your diet; remove all foods you may be sensitive to from your diet. Make sure you avoid sugars and greasy or fried foods.
2. Wash your skin and your hands frequently, but not enough to create skin sensitivity or abrasions from the washing or scrubbing.
3. Use over-the-counter products containing benzoyl peroxide (2.5%) or salicylic acid to dry up the acne and prevent new breakouts. Use these products carefully, and make sure to report any unwanted effects to your doctor. Be careful with any medication to avoid sun exposure and to avoid foods that interact with any medication.
4. Make sure you understand when you need professional help from a qualified doctor for your acne. You should see a doctor if you have acne that does not respond to your home treatments, and if you are concerned that you may get permanent scarring from your acne, or you have deep cystic acne that stops you or prevents you from wanted social activities.
5. Once you make the decision to visit your doctor, go with specific goals in mind. Let your doctor know what you want and stay committed to the plan. Do everything he/she prescribes for you, and make sure you know when to move to the next treatment. Isotretinoin or Accutane is usually a last resort drug and should be used only if you understand ***all of the risks!***

Action Plan for Eczema

1. Define the type of eczema you have. The more you know about your type, the better your chances will be of getting results without wasting time and money.
2. Take care of your skin daily. Wear softer clothes that don't scratch or irritate your skin, and use lotions or creams to soothe your skin. Don't take baths or showers that are too hot, or use soaps that irritate, as these will cause more problems for your skin.
3. Alter your diet, if necessary. Many people with eczema find that eliminating dairy and grain from their diet helps their skin. You may also find that getting rid of animals and carpets in your environment will also help, because many people are allergic or sensitive to pet dander or synthetic fibers in carpet.
4. Avoid sudden changes in temperature, and use a humidifier in the winter to prevent additional drying of your skin.
5. As simple as it sounds, don't scratch your skin—and trim the nails of children with eczema to prevent infections or skin breakdown from scratching.

Action Plan for Psoriasis

1. Again, you need to identify what type of psoriasis you have to make sure you get the right type of care. There are many types of psoriasis; your diagnosis needs to be made by a ***doctor who specializes in dermatology!***
2. Take daily baths to remove the excess skin, use moisturizers, cover the plaqued areas of skin at night, and make sure you avoid triggers and expose your skin to small amounts of sunlight. Try topical over-the-counter medications first. Always stop any medication that causes a rash or itching on any part of your body. (https://www.psoriasis.org/sublearn03_mild_otc)
3. You will also want to avoid drinking alcohol and you must eat a healthy diet to lessen your symptoms. You may also want to consider adding aloe vera and fish oil to your diet to help with the inflammation of your skin. We have patients who report that a gluten-free diet helps!
4. If you don't get relief from your psoriasis with creams and moisturizers, or over-the-counter medications that contain steroids and anti-itch ingredients, then move on to prescription medications recommended by a dermatologist.
5. Last, you will need a dermatologist who may prescribe phototherapy or laser treatment, and then ingested or injected medications, to help your symptoms. Retinoids, methotrexate, cyclosporine, hydroxyurea, and immunomodulators are used, and all have different side effects you must be aware of to lessen the chance of complications from their use. (http://www.mayoclinic.com/health/psoriasis/DS00193/DSECTION=treatments-and-drugs)

Action Plan for Skin Cancer

1. Avoid the sun during the mid-day and wear protective clothing or sun-screen to lessen your exposure.
2. Make sure you know when you are using medications that may make your skin more sensitive to the sun (common photo-toxic drugs are the tetracycline family, NSAIDs [non-steroidal anti-inflammatory drugs such as ibuprofen], and amiodarone, a heart medication). (http://www.webmd.com/skin-problems-and-treatments/sun-sensitizing-drugs)
3. Check your skin regularly and have someone else check areas you cannot see. Report directly to your doctor any changes you see as soon as you see changes in the area, or if you experience any of the problems listed above.
4. The earlier you go to the doctor, the less surgery you are likely to need! Small lesions don't usually require surgery, so if you think a spot may be cancerous, don't delay your care, ***it won't go away on its own!***
5. If you get bad news, follow your doctor's recommendations exactly! There are a lot of times I would tell you to try other ways to heal your body, but when it comes to cancer (or something that might be), I will tell you to please get professional advice and help!

Action Plan for High Cholesterol

1. The first step to getting your cholesterol under control is recognizing that you may have a problem and getting your blood tested. Then, know your cholesterol numbers and set a realistic goal of where you want to be!
2. Clean up your diet. Eat less red meat, way less fried food, more fish and chicken, and as many (raw) veggies as you can! These steps alone will help you lower your LDL.
3. Exercise every day, if you can. You don't need to turn yourself into a gym rat (although it wouldn't hurt), but get about thirty minutes of exercise per day and make sure you ***don't overdo!***
4. If you smoke, STOP! Smoking and being overweight are the one-two punch to your heart, and high cholesterol will add fuel to the fire. If you want to try some natural products which seem to help, try red rice yeast, which is a natural source of statins.
5. If you try everything above and your cholesterol is still out of range, you probably have genetic factors which drive your cholesterol. This may mean you may need to resort to medication to get your numbers down. Read the research and make sure you understand the risks of any medicine you use before taking the medicine!

Action Plan for Anxiety

1. The first step to treating yourself is to find out how anxiety affects you! A short pencil is better than a long memory, so write your feelings and thoughts down! Remember how anxiety affects you, what you feel, who is involved in your stress, and when you feel it. Then write down what you want from your life and how this problem stops you from getting it!
2. If you are going to try to treat yourself first (which I suggest), ask others if they have the same problems and feelings and get some input about how to start. Get simple, honest advice and don't share with anyone who may not care about you or who isn't interested in your success!
3. Learn how to help yourself. ***Do not allow negative self-talk to exist or continue!*** I have caught myself thousands of times speaking hatefully to me! When this happens, start over and see if you can find a way to change the way you talk to yourself. Focus on the things you are good at, and work to improve your strengths! You may still have some weaknesses, but don't focus on them as much! There are many millionaire athletes who stink at one part of a game, but they are millionaires because their strengths outshine their weaknesses.
4. Take time for you! Meditate, exercise, rest, and do everything you can to stop yourself from getting too stressed out. Remember that stress can be used as a motivator, and use it for that purpose only. You are in control of everything in your life until you give your control away!
5. If you try everything, or think you may need help to overcome your anxiety, get help! The longer you wait to treat your anxiety, the harder it is to get it under control. Learn your options before going to the doctor or therapist, and make wise choices about

your care. (http://www.medicalnewstoday.com/info/anxiety/anxiety-treatments)

Action Plan for Mental Problems

1. Determine which type of problems you are dealing with and move ***quickly*** to get the help necessary for the person you love or yourself. ***Never attempt to treat yourself!*** Many times people are wrong about the type of mental problem/s, and they diagnose themselves wrong!
2. Remember exercise and diet are factors that affect everything. Get the best food you can afford, and exercise regularly to help manage the problem/s. Understand that mental health is critical to your well-being, and care may be a lifetime event.
3. A psychologist and a psychiatrist do similar things, but ***are not the same!*** Both may refer you to another type of professional to help the problem, but the psychiatrist may be better suited to your needs if you need medication to manage the symptoms of your disease. Make your choice for care and follow the recommendations of your care-giver exactly for the best results!
4. Family members should be included in therapy, if at all possible. You will need a strong support structure for your therapy to succeed. This means you may need to exclude those people close to you who are not committed to your health and well-being. Look at tendencies in those who may have these problems; family problems and abuse may lead to mental problems in adulthood.
5. Never change or stop your therapy without the direction and consent of your chosen medical provider. The results could be disastrous and/or dangerous.

Action Plan to Slow Alzheimer's

1. Current research shows that there are many factors that contribute to Alzheimer's. Your age, the genes you inherit, where you live and work, your lifestyle, and any medical problems you may have may affect how and when Alzheimer's will strike, or if it will strike you at all. ***The only two you can't control are age and genetics. The rest can be influenced to help you lessen your chances for Alzheimer's.***
2. Unfortunately, there are no treatments (drug treatments) that work to stop Alzheimer's, and there are no tests that will give you an accurate warning (yet). However, as medicine advances, we may soon have tests and/or treatments that will be of some use to Alzheimer's victims.
3. Remember the connection between your heart and your brain! When you think of Alzheimer's, think of the things you may do that affect your heart. Because your brain gets nutrition from your blood, anything that hurts your heart will also hurt your brain! Some studies have shown that up to 80% of people diagnosed with Alzheimer's also had heart disease! This may mean that even with the tangles and plaques found in the brain during the disease, the disease may not be as bad (and/or may not develop) if there is no heart disease in the patient.
4. Physical exercise and diet are vitally important to help your circulation and nourish your brain. Diet and exercise decrease heart-related disease and stop plaque from developing in your blood vessels. A Mediterranean diet, which reduces red meat and focuses on whole grains, fruits and vegetables, seafood, olive oil and nuts, is a good way to begin for most people. Exercise to get your heart beating will also help keep your blood vessels clear.

5. Make sure you do not hit your head or suffer unnecessary head trauma. This may sound like fairly obvious advice, but head trauma can cause damage to the brain which will only make Alzheimer's worse. Anything that would negatively impact your brain should be avoided at all costs. If you love contact sports, or snow skiing or boarding, always wear a helmet!
6. Maintain social interaction and keep learning. Since one of the signs of Alzheimer's is a loss of social contacts and loss of memory, it only makes good sense to keep learning and keep interacting with others. This forces your brain to maintain connections and pathways that may otherwise be destroyed! (http://www.alz.org/research/science/alzheimers_prevention_and_risk.asp)
7. Make sure you monitor your progress with a professional and keep tabs on how your medicines work for you! We found that standard use of the prescribed medicines for our family member did not work as hoped, and her medications had to be adjusted to give her better results.
8. Make sure you have planned for all outcomes! Give specific directions to anyone who is given medical power of attorney for your care if you become unable to make decisions for yourself.
9. Keep up with current treatments! Medicine makes new discoveries every year. A new drug therapy or a new treatment may offer help in the near future, so keep searching online for any help.

Action Plan for High Blood Pressure

1. Know what kind of high blood pressure you have. Check your blood pressure daily, before you have any coffee or tea. We ask our patients to check their blood pressure first thing in the morning to get a baseline.
2. If your blood pressure is high, know your numbers! Remember, 120/80 is your goal unless you have other diseases which complicate your health and make this number unrealistic. Take your medication regularly and at the same time each day. Ask your doctor if you can take your medicine at night if it keeps you from sleeping (waking up to pee can cost you valuable sleep). Remember, the new guidelines as you age mean you may have blood pressure of up to 150/90 if you are older than 60 with no health problems.
3. Get your weight under control by eating right and begin a doctor-approved exercise program. Make sure you include your doctor in any decisions you make to change your health, especially if you decide to discontinue a prescribed medicine for any reason!
4. Understand how your medicines work and make sure you tell your doctor ***all of the medicines you take and what they are for!*** Be aware of any and all drug interactions and side effects.
5. If your blood pressure remains high, even if you are taking your medicines regularly, you must go to the doctor for help! High blood pressure can cause major damage to the organs in your body, and can cause a stroke which could kill you! Don't let any of these problems develop by failing to get needed help.

Action plan for Headaches

1. First, you must determine the type of headache you have. Once you have decided the type, look at the treatments you may use and get busy! The first step in treating headaches is always to see if there is an underlying allergy or food sensitivity. If there is, eliminate the food or substance and see if your headaches stop. Then, move on to the next treatment or try a combination of natural therapies before moving on to drug treatments. Remember that gluten is common in a lot of foods and elimination of gluten has helped many people with headaches.
2. The second step is to reduce your stress levels and try massage or chiropractic. I would try all of the easy things **before** you start any drug therapy. Acupuncture is next if you don't like the massage or chiropractic option. Remember to look at small things like drinking (coffee or alcohol), your posture, and sleeping and work positions! These may add to the mechanical stress and cause headaches.
3. Drug therapy should ***always*** begin with over-the-counter drugs! See if plain aspirin will help with your headaches (make sure you are not allergic and do not have ulcers), or try white willow bark if you prefer the more natural option. Move on to the over-the-counter antihistamines, and remember to avoid any drugs that do not work with medicine you already take.
4. Step four is to go to the doctor for help with other drugs. Tell your doctor all ***of your symptoms!*** Include what you have already tried (written form is better) and the results. Make sure you understand the medicines he prescribes and the side effects you may experience.
5. Now you need to consider the most aggressive therapies to treat your headaches: trigger point injections, Botox injections, elec-

trode implants (if your headaches are disabling), or a mix of therapies to get rid of your headaches. I hope you never need this step, but many people find help in this last step

Action Plan for Diabetes

1. Recognize the early signs of diabetes. Type I (juvenile) diabetes usually affects younger people and causes weight loss. Type II diabetes is called "adult onset diabetes" and may cause weight gain.
2. Understand that diabetes may affect your entire body and develop an action plan for dealing with the disease. The first step should be to get your blood work done and make sure that your doctor checks your thyroid! Make sure you understand how your thyroid may drive diabetes, and if this is an issue for you, correct the thyroid first.
3. Learn everything you can about nutrition. The main way to curb diabetes in most people is with proper nutrition. Eliminate empty calories from sugar and foods that convert quickly to sugar (rice, potatoes, bread and pasta). Try eliminating gluten from your diet to help your thyroid and remove toxins from your body.
4. If your diabetes does not respond to these steps, go to the doctor! You will need the advice of an endocrinologist. He/she may be able to help you treat your diabetes without drugs…if you get into the office early enough!
5. Remember that diabetes can be deadly. ***Never*** try to treat yourself by using medication that your doctor did not prescribe, and never stop taking medication without telling your doctor. Many people have died trying to self-regulate a medication (taking medicine only when they feel bad, even when the doctor tells them they need the medicine).

Final Thoughts

I hope you get everything you want out of this life. I have had the good fortune to live my dream and love my life (for the most part). If you want to live the life you dream of, make the changes that will help you make your dreams come true.

Most people will never make the cover of *Cosmo* or be a *GQ* guy or a Victoria's Secret girl. You don't need to be famous to have a magical life. But you do need good health to enjoy life to its fullest! Even if you have a disease, it doesn't mean you can't be happy, productive, and make a difference on this planet.

I have seen videos of people born with disfigurements and disabilities that I would hate who are more productive and happier than most people I know who could be classed as "high achievers." Your mind is more powerful than you know.

Now you have the information to help yourself. If you would like me to write more information on any topic, let me know. I'd love to help people the world over get better and do better. It's my passion to make the world a healthier, better place for everyone, and education is the key!

Cheers and great health!
David Bush

www.ingramcontent.com/pod-product-compliance
Lightning Source LLC
Chambersburg PA
CBHW060843280326
41934CB00007B/896

* 9 7 8 0 9 8 6 1 2 5 4 8 5 *